Video Capsule Endoscopy

Editor

DAVID R. CAVE

GASTROINTESTINAL ENDOSCOPY CLINICS OF NORTH AMERICA

www.giendo.theclinics.com

Consulting Editor
CHARLES J. LIGHTDALE

April 2021 • Volume 31 • Number 2

ELSEVIER

1600 John F. Kennedy Boulevard • Suite 1800 • Philadelphia, Pennsylvania, 19103-2899

http://www.theclinics.com

GASTROINTESTINAL ENDOSCOPY CLINICS OF NORTH AMERICA Volume 31, Number 2
April 2021 ISSN 1052-5157, ISBN-13: 978-0-323-79618-7

Editor: Kerry Holland
Developmental Editor: Donald Mumford

Gastrointestinal Endoscopy Clinics of North America (ISSN 1052-5157) is published quarterly by Elsevier Inc., 360 Park Avenue South, New York, NY 10010-1710. Months of issue are January, April, July, and October. Business and Editorial Offices: 1600 John F. Kennedy Blvd., Suite 1800, Philadelphia, PA, 19103-2899. Periodicals postage paid at New York, NY and additional mailing offices. Subscription prices are $363.00 per year for US individuals, $813.00 per year for US institutions, $100.00 per year for US and Canadian students/residents, $399.00 per year for Canadian individuals, $841.00 per year for Canadian institutions, $476.00 per year for international individuals, $841.00 per year for international institutions, and $245.00 per year for international students/residents. To receive student/resident rate, orders must be accompanied by name of affiliated institution, date of term, and the *signature* of program/residency coordinator on institution letterhead. Orders will be billed at individual rate until proof of status is received. Foreign air speed delivery is included in all *Clinics* subscription prices. All prices are subject to change without notice. **POSTMASTER:** Send address change to *Gastrointestinal Endoscopy Clinics of North America*, Elsevier Health Sciences Division, Subscription Customer Service, 3251 Riverport Lane, Maryland Heights, MO 63043. **Customer Service: 1-800-654-2452 (US). From outside the United States, call 1-314-447-8871. Fax: 1-314-447-8029. E-mail: JournalsCustomerService-usa@elsevier.com (for print support) or JournalsOnlineSupport-usa@elsevier.com (for online support).**

Reprints. For copies of 100 or more, of articles in this publication, please contact the Commercial Reprints Department, Elsevier Inc., 360 Park Avenue South, New York, NY 10010-1710. Tel. 212-633-3874; Fax: 212-633-3820; E-mail: reprints@elsevier.com.

Gastrointestinal Endoscopy Clinics of North America is covered in *Excerpta Medica, MEDLINE/PubMed (Index Medicus), and MEDLINE/MEDLARS.*

Contributors

CONSULTING EDITOR

CHARLES J. LIGHTDALE, MD
Professor of Medicine, Division of Digestive and Liver Diseases, Columbia University, Medical Center, New York, New York, USA

EDITOR

DAVID R. CAVE, MD, PhD, FACG
Professor of Medicine, University of Massachusetts, Director of Clinical Gastroenterology Research, Division of Gastroenterology, Department of Medicine, University of Massachusetts Medical School, UMass Memorial Medical Center, Worcester, Massachusetts, USA

AUTHORS

DOUGLAS G. ADLER, MD
University of Utah School of Medicine, Salt Lake City, Utah, USA

JACQUELYN G. BOLWELL, MD
Medical Instructor, Department of Medicine, Duke University Medical Center, Durham, North Carolina, USA

MAURO BRUNO, MD
University Division of Gastroenterology, City of Health and Science University Hospital, Turin, Italy

DAVID R. CAVE, MD, PhD, FACG
Professor of Medicine, University of Massachusetts, Director of Clinical Gastroenterology Research, Division of Gastroenterology, Department of Medicine, University of Massachusetts Medical School, UMass Memorial Medical Center, Worcester, Massachusetts, USA

LAUREL R. FISHER, MD
Professor of Clinical Medicine, Director, Small Bowel Imaging Program, Division of Gastroenterology and Hepatology, University of Pennsylvania Health System, Philadelphia, Pennsylvania, USA

SHRADHA GUPTA, MD
Department of Medicine, University of Massachusetts Medical School, Worcester, Massachusetts, USA

SHAHRAD HAKIMIAN, MD
Gastroenterology Fellow, Department of Medicine, Division of Gastroenterology, University of Massachusetts Medical School, Worcester, Massachusetts, USA

MARK HANSCOM, MD
Gastroenterology Fellow, Department of Medicine, Division of Gastroenterology, University of Massachusetts Medical School, UMass Memorial Medical Center, Worcester, Massachusetts, USA

ARIOSTO HERNANDEZ-LARA, MD
Research Fellow, Developmental Endoscopy Unit, Mayo Clinic, Rochester, Minnesota, USA

LAWRENCE HOOKEY, MD, FRCP(C), FCAG
Gastrointestinal Diseases Research Unit, Department of Medicine, Queen's University, Professor, Division of Gastroenterology, Hotel Dieu Hospital, Kingston, Ontario, Canada

SALMAAN JAWAID, MD
Assistant Professor of Medicine, Gastroenterology-Advanced Endoscopy, Baylor College of Medicine, Houston, Texas, USA

ANASTASIOS KOULAOUZIDIS, MD, MD(Res), PhD, FEBG
Department of Gastroenterology, Royal Infirmary of Edinburgh, Edinburgh, Scotland

JOEL LANGE, MD
Department of Emergency Medicine, George Washington University School of Medicine and Health Sciences, Washington, DC, USA

JONATHAN A. LEIGHTON, MD
Vice Chair, Department of Internal Medicine, Professor of Medicine, College of Medicine, Mayo Clinic, Scottsdale, Arizona, USA

NEIL B. MARYA, MD
Assistant Professor of Clinical Medicine, Division of Gastroenterology, University of Massachusetts Medical School, Worcester, Massachusetts, USA

JOSIAH D. McCAIN, MD
Fellow, Division of Gastroenterology and Hepatology, Mayo Clinic, Scottsdale, Arizona, USA

ANDREW C. MELTZER, MD, MS
Associate Professor, Department of Emergency Medicine, George Washington University School of Medicine and Health Sciences, Washington, DC, USA

DEJAN MICIC, MD
Assistant Professor of Medicine, Department of Internal Medicine, Section of Gastroenterology, Hepatology and Nutrition, University of Chicago, Chicago, Illinois, USA

SHABANA F. PASHA, MD
Vice Chair, Division of Gastroenterology and Hepatology, Professor of Medicine, College of Medicine, Mayo Clinic, Scottsdale, Arizona, USA

MARCO PENNAZIO, MD
University Division of Gastroenterology, City of Health and Science University Hospital, Turin, Italy

PATRICK D. POWERS
Department of Medicine, University of Massachusetts Medical School, Worcester, Massachusetts, USA

DANIEL L. RAINES, MD
New Orleans, Louisiana, USA

ELIZABETH RAJAN, MD, FASGE
Consultant Gastroenterologist and Professor of Medicine, Division of Gastroenterology
and Hepatology, Mayo Clinic, Rochester, Minnesota, USA

MICHELLE RICCI, MD, FRCP(C)
Gastrointestinal Diseases Research Unit, Department of Medicine, Queen's University,
Kingston, Ontario, Canada

ALEXANDER ROSS ROBERTSON, MBChB, MRCP, AFHEA
Department of Gastroenterology, Western General Hospital, Edinburgh, Scotland

EMANUELE RONDONOTTI, MD, PhD
Gastroenterology Unit, Valduce Hospital, Como, Italy

CAROL E. SEMRAD, MD
Professor of Medicine, Department of Internal Medicine, Section of Gastroenterology,
Hepatology and Nutrition, University of Chicago, Chicago, Illinois, USA

AROOJ SHAH, MD
Department of Emergency Medicine, George Washington Medical Faculty Associates,
Washington, DC, USA

ANUPAM SINGH, MD
Assistant Professor, Division of Gastroenterology, UMass Memorial Medical Center,
North Worcester, Massachusetts, USA

ELIZABETH SQUIRELL, MD, FRCP(C)
Gastrointestinal Diseases Research Unit, Department of Medicine, Queen's University,
Kingston, Ontario, Canada

PETER SULLIVAN, MD
Department of Medicine, University of Massachusetts Medical School, Worcester,
Massachusetts, USA

DANIEL WILD, MD
Associate Professor of Medicine, Associate Clinical Chief, Director of Small Bowel
Endoscopy, Division of Gastroenterology, Duke University Medical Center, Durham,
North Carolina, USA

RICHARD M. WU, MD, MPH
Assistant Professor of Clinical Medicine, Division of Gastroenterology and Hepatology,
Corporal Michael J. Crescenz Veterans Affairs Medical Center, University of Pennsylvania
Health System, Philadelphia, Pennsylvania, USA

Contents

Video capsule endoscopy (VCE) is an established modality for examining the small bowel. Formal training in interpretation and reporting of VCE examinations, along with assessment of performance metrics, is advocated for all gastroenterology fellowship programs. This review provides an overview of VCE minimum training requirements and competency assessment, cognitive and technical aspects of interpretation, and standardized reporting of findings. In order to optimize and advance the clinical utility of VCE, efforts must continue to promote and encourage consensus and standardization of training, definition and assessment of competence, enhancements of VCE reading tools, and use of appropriate nomenclature in VCE reports.

There is a trend in data to support active preparation for video capsule endoscopy (VCE), but the timing of this remains unclear. Split dosing may be the most efficacious preparation. Study methodology continues to evolve, with increased use of standardized scales, with the addition of diagnostic yield as an outcome. The use of adjuncts has not been detrimental, but their value has not been proved to improve outcomes of VCE.

Video capsule endoscopy is indicated in a broad range of clinical settings, most commonly in evaluating suspected small bowel bleeding. It is also useful in diagnosing Crohn's disease and monitoring patients with known Crohn's. Video capsule endoscopy has a role in evaluating patients with refractory celiac disease symptoms and in surveying patients with polyposis syndromes. The only absolute contraindication to video capsule endoscopy is luminal gastrointestinal tract obstruction. Despite manufacturer statement, video capsule endoscopy can be used safely in patients with implantable cardiac devices including pacemakers, defibrillators, and ventricular assist devices.

Video capsule endoscopy has an essential role in the diagnosis and management of small bowel bleeding and is the first-line study recommended for this purpose. This article reviews the risk factors for small bowel bleeding, optimal timing for video capsule endoscopy testing, and algorithms recommended for evaluation. Used primarily for the assessment of nonacute gastrointestinal blood loss, video capsule endoscopy has an emerging role for more urgent use in emergency settings and in special populations. Future software incorporation of neural networks to enhance lesion detection will likely result in an augmented role of video capsule endoscopy in small bowel bleeding.

Video capsule endoscopy (VCE) is a crucial adjunct to conventional endoscopy in small intestinal bleeding, with a high positive and negative predictive value. Timing is critical in VCE, with earlier deployment associated with improved diagnostic yield. VCE is also useful as a first-line diagnostic modality in the evaluation of acute gastrointestinal bleeding, with accumulating evidence demonstrating expedited VCE can increase diagnostic yield, reduce unneeded admissions, and overall improve patient care. In resource-limited settings, first-line VCE also can reduce unneeded procedures and protect staff from dangerous exposures.

 Video content accompanies this article at http://www.giendo. theclinics.com.

The cause of small intestinal bleeding (SIB) may be elusive despite exhaustive testing. This article describes the current understanding of SIB regarding evaluation, with emphasis on the use of video capsule endoscopy (VCE) as a diagnostic procedure. This article addresses the utility of provocative testing in challenging cases and the performance of endoscopic procedures on active antithrombotic therapy. Specific recommendations accompany this article, including use of antithrombotic agents to stimulate bleeding when clearly indicated; performance of endoscopic procedures on active antithrombotic therapy; and progressive adoption of VCE and device-assisted enteroscopy in the inpatient setting.

 Video content accompanies this article at http://www.giendo. theclinics.com.

Video capsule endoscopy and device-assisted enteroscopy are complementary technologies. Capsule endoscopy is a highly acceptable technology with high diagnostic yield that can guide a subsequent entero-scopy approach. This article aims to focus on the role of video capsule endoscopy as a prelude to deep enteroscopy with a focus on the strengths and limitations of either approach.

 Video content accompanies this article at http://www.giendo. theclinics.com.

In Crohn disease (CD), the use of capsule endoscopy (CE) for suspected versus established disease is very different. Most patients with CD are diagnosed with ileocolonoscopy. In patients with a negative ileocolono-scopy, CE is the next best test in suspected CD. In patients with estab-lished CD, the potential benefits of CE are rating severity of disease, establishing extent and distribution, and following mucosal healing in a treat to target strategy. In those with proximal small bowel disease, CE can help in diagnosis and prognostication. In ulcerative colitis, CE has a limited role, but that may change with evolving technology.

 Video content accompanies this article at http://www.giendo. theclinics.com.

In the setting of chronic liver disease, capsule endoscopy is safe and well tolerated, making it an appealing diagnostic procedure. It is used mainly for the surveillance of esophageal varices, investigation of anemia, and exploration of the small bowel for complications of portal hypertension. Capsule endoscopy is recognized as a viable alternative in patients unable or unwilling to undergo upper gastrointestinal endoscopy for investigations of esophageal varices. In evaluating the small bowel of patients with liver disease and unexplained anemia, capsule endoscopy increases recogni-tion of mucosal abnormalities, although their clinical significance is often unclear.

Video capsule endoscopy has been proven to be a beneficial tool to inspect the gastrointestinal lumen but its true impact may lie in utilization outside of traditional gastroenterology settings such as in the emergency room, the intensive care unit, and outpatient settings. Some advantages of video capsule endoscopy are that its administration does not require special training, patients do not require anesthesia, and videos can be shared with off-site consultants.

Artificial intelligence (AI) research for medical applications has expanded quickly. Advancements in computer processing now allow for the development of complex neural network architectures (eg, convolutional neural networks) that are capable of extracting and learning complex features from massive data sets, including large image databases. Gastroenterology and endoscopy are well suited for AI research. Video capsule endoscopy is an ideal platform for AI model research given the large amount of data produced by each capsule examination and the annotated databases that are already available. Studies have demonstrated high performance for applications of capsule-based AI models developed for various pathologic conditions.

 Video content accompanies this article at http://www.giendo. theclinics.com.

Video capsule endoscopy is entering its third decade. After slow acceptance, it has become the gold standard in diagnosing small intestinal disorders. This article summarizes new practical applications for capsule endoscopy outside the small intestine. From 2 randomized controlled trials, it is becoming clear that it has a role in the management of patients with hematemesis and nonhematemesis bleeding. Under active investigation are novel applications of capsule technology, including the potential ability to sample luminal contents or tissue, self-propelled capsules, incorporation of other imaging techniques beyond white light, such as ultrasound and fluorescents, and the possibility of drug delivery.

The development of video capsule endoscopy (VCE) has allowed for visualization of parts of the gastrointestinal tract generally not readily accessible by noninvasive means. Its ease of use has proved useful in diagnosing and managing various small bowel inflammatory disorders. Continued technological evolution of VCE has paved the way for use in small intestinal bleeding and in patients with acute gastrointestinal bleeding. A detailed analysis of costs associated with VCE has demonstrated its ability to promote efficient allocation of health care resources. Further work is needed regarding development of a universal infrastructure to handle the widespread use of VCE technology.

GASTROINTESTINAL ENDOSCOPY CLINICS OF NORTH AMERICA

RELATED CLINICS SERIES

Gastroenterology Clinics
(www.gastro.theclinics.com)
Clinics in Liver Disease
(www.liver.theclinics.com)

THE CLINICS ARE AVAILABLE ONLINE!
Access your subscription at:
www.theclinics.com

Foreword

Video Capsule Endoscopy: Safe, Effective, Evolving, Here to Stay

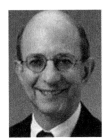

Charles J. Lightdale, MD
Consulting Editor

It's interesting when a completely new technology arrives on the scene in gastrointestinal endoscopy. There are always the doubters, the head scratchers, the worriers, and then the early adopters and pioneers, who become essential to potential success. Two decades ago, video capsule endoscopy was a completely new technology: a tiny video camera, transmitter, and battery jammed into a pill-sized cylinder that could be swallowed by most people, and easily pass through the entire gastrointestinal tract. The main target organ was the small intestine, the last and most difficult frontier for gastrointestinal endoscopists to examine completely.

David R. Cave, the Editor for this issue of the *Gastrointestinal Endoscopy Clinics of North America* dedicated entirely to video capsule endoscopy, was an early adopter, who saw the potential for the noninvasive technology to identify small bowel abnormalities otherwise very difficult to detect by other methods. Dr Cave was the Editor for an issue of the *Gastrointestinal Endoscopy Clinics of North America* in 2009 devoted to endoscopic examination of the small intestine (enteroscopy), which highlighted the growing utilization of the video capsule approach. Now, a dozen years later, it seemed a great time to invite him back as Editor for this issue. He has selected an extraordinary group of experts to compile an array of topics that define the state-of-the-art of video capsule endoscopy and a look at its evolution and future. There are very practical topics covered, including training, reading, and reporting for small bowel cases, and how to improve results using preparation, timing, prokinetics, and surface-active agents. A full discussion of growing indications and a few notable contraindications are presented. The role of video capsule endoscopy in the diagnosis and localization of small intestinal bleeding is covered thoroughly, including an article on the timing and use of video capsule endoscopy in the acute care setting. Another important topic explores the role of video capsule endoscopy as a prelude to deep enteroscopy, and other articles describe the utility of the capsule in inflammatory bowel disease and liver disease.

Gastrointest Endoscopy Clin N Am 31 (2021) xiii–xiv
https://doi.org/10.1016/j.giec.2021.01.003
1052-5157/21/© 2021 Published by Elsevier Inc.
giendo.theclinics.com

Certainly, the optics and imaging of video capsule endoscopy have improved tremendously in recent years, but despite improvements in software, reading the small bowel examinations can still be tedious and time consuming. Artificial intelligence has great promise to improve this problem, and research and development in AI for video capsule endoscopy is presented. Looking to the future, in another article are additional technical developments that tickle the imagination and offer the possibility of novel clinical applications. Finally, coming back to earth, there is a key discussion of the cost-effectiveness of video capsule endoscopy, so critical to present to hospital and practice administrators, who must decide on purchasing the needed capsules and equipment. This issue of the *Gastrointestinal Endoscopy Clinics of North America* should convince almost everyone that video capsule endoscopy is here to stay.

Charles J. Lightdale, MD
Department of Medicine
Columbia University Medical Center
161 Fort Washington Avenue
New York, NY 10032, USA

E-mail address:
cjl18@cumc.columbia.edu

Preface

Video Capsule Endoscopy: Now and the Future

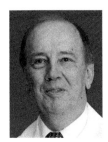

David R. Cave, MD, PhD
Editor

My first interaction with video capsule endoscopy was in early 2001, when I was invited to a marketing focus group run on behalf of a startup company by the name of Given Imaging (Yokneam, Israel). The little pill-like device that was demonstrated took rather fuzzy low-resolution images of the small intestine from pylorus to ileocecal valve. This was to be an answer to a prayer. I and a few others had been struggling with different ways to access the small bowel for more than a decade, particularly for people who had small intestinal bleeding. We had tried with Sonde enteroscopy, push enteroscopy, and intraoperative enteroscopy. None of these were very satisfactory. They were very time consuming, particularly the Sonde enteroscope, which could take all day for peristalsis to drag the small balloon on the tip of many feet of fiber-optic cable, all or partially along the length of the small intestine, and, which on withdrawal, might provide a transient image of an angioectasia.

By August 2001, the Food and Drug Administration had approved the M_2A capsule as a result of the pivotal trial conducted on 25 patients by Blair Lewis and Paul Swain. I had previously contacted Given Imaging and was given a small grant to start using the capsule in patients. This little device revealed a treasure trove of pathologic condition in the small intestine in a manner not seen before. It was reminiscent of the film "A Fantastic Voyage." At the time, the device evoked more media attention than professional attention, but, over time, this has slowly changed. Nearly 20 years later, there are 4 approved devices in the United States, 2 in China, and others around the world. The focus has been predominantly on the small intestine, and its slow, but revolutionary evolution, at least in part, is due to the long reading time that may be involved.

With the help of some of the world's leading capsule endoscopists, I have been able to compile an issue that contains up-to-the-minute clinical science on many aspects of the utilization of video capsule endoscopy. My hope is that this will provide a valuable

https://doi.org/10.1016/j.giec.2021.01.002
1052-5157/21/© 2021 Published by Elsevier Inc.

giendo.theclinics.com

resource for trainees, established practitioners, faculty, and the greater scientific community.

The articles in the issue by Robertson and colleagues and Lange and colleagues are devoted to avenues of advancement of technology as applied to capsule endoscopy. Artificial intelligence has already started to impact the field and provides a solution to the problem of the tedium of reading and will probably prove to be more accurate, particularly for patients who have an abnormality on a single frame that is so easy to miss. The article by Micic and the article by Jawaid discuss applications of capsule endoscopy outside the small intestine that are beginning to appear, and new devices that may be able to be externally controlled by a magnetic field, self-propelled, take a biopsy, and or to deliver drugs. From the patient's point of view, capsule endoscopy is very appealing, as it is noninvasive and currently has application in the esophagus, stomach, duodenum, and colon for a wide range of different conditions.

Over the next decade, it is not difficult to conceive of video capsule endoscopy being used much more widely and starting to erode the role of conventional endoscopy to the benefit of our patients. It is not difficult to envisage interrogation of the entire gastrointestinal tract either locally at the site of deployment, as is done now, or remotely in the future.

David R. Cave, MD, PhD
Division of Gastroenterology
Department of Medicine
University of Massachusetts
UMass Memorial Medical Center
55 Lake Avenue North
Worcester, MA 01655, USA

E-mail address:
david.cave@umassmemorial.org

Training, Reading, and Reporting for Small Bowel Video Capsule Endoscopy

Ariosto Hernandez-Lara, MD[a], Elizabeth Rajan, MD[b],*

KEYWORDS

- Capsule endoscopy • Training • Evaluation • Competency • Reading • Reporting
- Guidelines

KEY POINTS

- Review of the evidence available on the impact of formalized video capsule endoscopy (VCE) training on achieving independent practice, and assessing competency.
- Define the cognitive and technical aspects of reading a VCE examination.
- Provide an update on standardized reporting of VCE findings.

INTRODUCTION

Video capsule endoscopy (VCE) is an established noninvasive modality for investigating small bowel disease and remains the diagnostic test of choice when evaluating small bowel bleeding.[1–15] With advances in VCE, a majority (approximately 75%) of patients previously classified as having obscure gastrointestinal bleeding are found to have a bleeding source within the small intestine.[2–4,11,15] Although VCE is widely used in clinical practice, there remains a lack of consensus and standardization on training, definition and assessment of competence, VCE reading protocol, and use of appropriate nomenclature when reporting VCE findings. Therefore, the aim of this review is to provide a comprehensive, current, and concise overview of VCE training requirements and assessment of competency; cognitive and technical aspects of interpretation; and standardized reporting of findings.

[a] Developmental Endoscopy Unit, Mayo Clinic, Rochester, MN, USA; [b] Division of Gastroenterology and Hepatology, Mayo Clinic, 200 First Street Southwest, Rochester, MN 55905, USA
* Corresponding author.
E-mail address: rajan.elizabeth16@mayo.edu

Gastrointest Endoscopy Clin N Am 31 (2021) 237–249
https://doi.org/10.1016/j.giec.2020.12.001

DISCUSSION
Training in Video Capsule Endoscopy

Guidelines and core curricula endorsed by national or international gastroenterology societies

American Society for Gastrointestinal Endoscopy. The American Society for Gastrointestinal Endoscopy (ASGE) guidelines for credentialing and granting of privileges to perform VCE recommend dedicated VCE training as part of a gastroenterology (GI) fellowship, or an 8-hour interactive continuing medical education (CME) course, followed by performance of 10 VCEs that are reviewed by a credentialed capsule endoscopist.[16] The ASGE Training Committee published an updated and comprehensive small bowel endoscopy core curriculum in 2013, recommending training programs provide formal lecture-based instructions and hands-on training in VCE during the 3-year GI fellowship.[17] When VCE training is unavailable during fellowship, trainees should complete a hands-on course with a minimum of 8 hours of CME credit, endorsed by a national or international GI society (eg, ASGE-sponsored VCE courses) followed by review of procedures by a credentialed capsule endoscopist. The core curriculum also highlights the need for trainees to have image recognition skills of normal and pathologic endoscopic findings acquired from performing upper endoscopy, colonoscopy, and push enteroscopy. Trainees should acquire a detailed knowledge of VCE indications, contraindications, informed consent, use of bowel preparation, and risks of capsule retention (including management) and magnetic resonance imaging. Trainees are expected to be familiar with the technical aspects of the VCE hardware and software, including the capsule delivery system and nonvideo patency capsule. Further emphasis is placed on programs that offer training in VCE to have sufficient volume, although this number remains unspecified, and on expert faculty committed to teaching VCE while providing timely feedback to trainees that includes integration of findings into a patient management plan.

Competency Assessment: a minimum of 20 procedures supervised by a credentialed capsule endoscopist are required while underscoring that proficiency should reflect competence and not numbers alone based on variability in individual learning curves. Passing a formalized in-service examination or achieving a 90% or greater correlation rate of significant findings compared with expert reader(s) is applied as a reasonable metric. In addition, competence should be determined by recording objective measures and direct observation by a qualified capsule endoscopist during training.

European Society of Gastrointestinal Endoscopy. In 2020, the European Society of Gastrointestinal Endoscopy (ESGE) published a detailed position statement on a curriculum for small bowel capsule endoscopy and device-assisted enteroscopy training in Europe.[18] The ESGE recommends that small bowel VCE courses consist of at least 50% hands-on training and include the technology, indications and contraindications, pathologies encountered, standard terminology to be used when reporting on VCE and formulation of an appropriate management plan for patients. Obtaining exposure to reading capsule studies is encouraged prior to a hands-on course. Experience in bidirectional endoscopies (upper endoscopy and colonoscopy) is recommended for training in VCE. The ESGE core curriculum provides criteria to be recognized as a training center that includes a minimum required volume of 75 to 100 small bowel VCEs per year and at least 1 faculty member to have reported on more than 500 studies and at least 1 faculty member to be experienced in device-assisted enteroscopy.

Competency assessment: a minimum of 30 supervised VCE reads are recommended in the absence of a structured assessment process. Direct observation of procedural skills, test videos, and multiple-choice questions can be useful to evaluate skills of trainees. Before achieving competence, a structured VCE training course/program should be completed.

Canadian Association of Gastroenterology. In 2017 the Canadian Association of Gastroenterology published guidelines recommending VCE be restricted to readers with documented competency in the cognitive and technical aspects of the procedure including reporting and interpreting VCE examinations.[19]

Competency assessment: the minimum number of VCE procedures required and parameters for competency assessment were not defined.

Current evidence
Training in video capsule endoscopy. Implementing a structured VCE training curriculum is advocated and recommended for all GI fellowship programs. An e-mail survey to GI fellowship program directors in the United States by Read and colleagues[20] had a 35.1% response rate (59 program directors responded) and indicated a promising 84.8% of GI programs required trainees to complete VCE training during their fellowship.

Limited evidence points to the beneficial outcomes of VCE training. A multicenter study on European courses found that trainees had improved diagnostic ability with capsule reading after attending courses with at least 50% hands-on training. Participants who had previous experience with 11 or more capsule studies before attending a structured hands-on course had higher baseline test scores for short videos.[21] Accuracy for pathologies, such as tumors and villous atrophy, was lower for trainees compared, with experts highlighting the importance of discussing common and rare entities during VCE courses.[22,23] Sidhu and colleagues[24] assessed the performance of 10 GI trainees and 5 medical students who reviewed 10 capsule studies with an expert. They found that previous endoscopic experience enabled readers to achieve a higher diagnostic accuracy. Rajan and colleagues[25,26] showed that the number of upper endoscopy, colonoscopy, push enteroscopy, or total endoscopy examinations performed by GI fellows did not have a significant association with VCE competence. These findings suggest that prior endoscopic experience and image recognition of normal and abnormal findings were important when training in VCE rather than the number of procedures performed.

Computer-based learning Structured e-learning platforms are an appealing alternative for VCE training. Postgate and colleagues[27] evaluated the effectiveness of a computer-based VCE training and testing module where GI trainees and medical students (n = 28) without VCE experience completed a 60-question module consisting of 30-second videos and multiple-choice questions. This study demonstrated significant improvement in lesion detection after training in both groups.

Competency assessment. A universally accepted VCE competency assessment tool is much needed. Based on the survey conducted by Read and colleagues,[20] a disappointing 3.4% of GI fellowship programs use some metric-based assessment tool. In 2006, Rajan and colleagues[26] developed and successfully implemented a structured VCE training curriculum in their GI fellowship program together with creating a formalized assessment tool, the capsule competency test (CapCT). A single-center 6-year prospective analysis of fellows' training and competence study was published, concluding that trainees should complete more than 20 VCE studies before assessing competence. In 2020, in order to determine if their single-center experience could be translated to other training programs, Rajan and colleagues[25] performed a prospective, multicenter study to determine the minimal threshold of VCE procedures required to achieve competence after a structured VCE training program and to validate the CapCT. This study concluded that GI fellows should complete a minimum of 25 supervised VCE interpretations before assessing competence using the validated CapCT, which had a high interobserver agreement among expert faculty (k = 0.85).[25]

A retrospective study by Velayos and colleagues,[28] assessing 900 VCE cases reviewed by 2 experts, found that the negative predictive values increased with number of cases reviewed but did not improve after the first 100 reads. A multicenter study from Europe showed a plateau in the learning curve for VCE after 25 procedures.[21] The Korean Gut Image Study Group found that competency of 12 trainees improved compared with experts after 9 capsule reads and 11 capsule reads (kappa >0.60 and >0.80, respectively).[29]

With the emerging evidence and guidelines available, the authors provide a summary on VCE training in **Table 1**. Training in VCE should be extended to nurses and other health care professionals who perform VCE prereads in some centers.

Reading a Video Capsule Endoscopy Examination

Interpretation of a VCE examination can be time consuming and may require between 30 minutes and 60 minutes to complete.[30] Tens of thousands of frames of images are acquired and analyzed carefully. Small bowel transit times (SBTTs) vary from 2 hours to 5 hours, and small bowel completion rates (cecal intubation) range from 78% to 100%.[31–33]

Reading times

Depending on the expertise of the reader and type of capsule system used, the frame rate for reviewing a VCE study generally is set between 10 frames/s and 20 frames/s. Reading at a slower rate runs the risk of losing focus and concentration with a more lengthy interpretation whereas higher reading rates can result in miss lesions.[34] No compromise in diagnostic yield between single-frame and multiframe viewing have been reported.[35–37] Innovative attempts have been made to incorporate automated smart software algorithms into commercially available capsule enteroscopy systems that discard redundant and repetitive images, resulting in VCE reads that are shorter while maintaining accuracy. Rapid reading software algorithms describe accuracies that range from 60% to 97%, with variations according to both the software used and clinical indication.[37–42] A further enhancement of the rapid reading software allows for sampling of select frames in order to create a shortened version of the VCE examination that can be reviewed in a few minutes (QuickView, RAPID Reader software, Minneapolis, Minnesota)[43–45] (**Table 2**). At this time, however, this abbreviated

Table 1 Training in video capsule endoscopy	
Pretraining	Experience in upper endoscopy, colonoscopy, and push enteroscopy
Training	1. Formal lecture-based instructions and hands-on training in VCE during GI fellowship *OR* 8 h of CME credit, endorsed by a national or international GI society 2. Direct observation of real-time cases of VCE interpretation by trainee 3. Completing at least 25 supervised interpretations of VCE examinations
Post-training	Metric-based competency assessment

Table 2
Small bowel capsule systems: rapid reading modes and times

Reference	Reading Mode/Company	Reading Time (Mean)	Number of Cases	Comparison to Conventional Mode
Kyriakos et al,[37] 2012	Automatic/PillCam SB2 (Medtronic, MN)	32.2 min	100	Miss rate: 1%
Beg et al,[38] 2020	Omni/EndoCapsule (Olympus, Tokyo, Japan)	17 min	315 (2127 lesions)	Accuracy: .75
Hosoe et al,[39] 2016	Omni/EndoCapsule (Olympus, Tokyo, Japan)	27.3 min	40	Not stated
Xu et al,[40] 2014	Similar picture elimination mode/OMOM (Jinshan Science and Technology Company, Chongqing, China)	24.9 min (level I)	200	Sensitivity: 87.7% Specificity: 98.5% (level I)
Saurin et al,[41] 2018	Express view/Mirocam (IntroMedic, Seoul, Republic of Korea)	19.7 min	83	Sensitivity: 82.2%
Pioche et al,[63] 2014	CapsoCam SV-1 (CapsoVision, Silicon Valley, CA)	32 min	73	Not applicable
Saurin et al,[44] 2012	QuickView/Pillcam SB2 (Medtronic, MN)	11.6 min	106	Sensitivity: 89.2% Specificity: 84% 8 missed lesions
Koulaouzidis et al,[43] 2012	QuickView/Pillcam SB2 (Medtronic, MN)	475 s	200	Sensitivity: 92.3% Specificity: 96.3%

version can be of help as a preview, especially in an urgent inpatient setting of small bowel bleeding, but should not replace the need to read an entire VCE study.

Suspected blood indicator and blue mode

The suspected blood indicator (SBI) is an informatic algorithm developed to select red-colored (blood) images or red pixels and correspondingly sets red bars as markers to alert the reader to the likely presence of blood. The SBI mode can be helpful particularly when quick and early identification of acute bleeding is required, for instance, in an in-patient or emergency room setting. A key limitation of the SBI function, however, is the presence of false-positive bars that often are related to bubbles or dark bile and not blood. Han and colleagues[46] performed a prospective validation of SBI to identify active small bowel bleeding in 100 patients, which demonstrated that, by using a cutoff of 8 contiguous, SBI markers there was 100% sensitivity and specificity in detecting blood. Tal and colleagues[47] created an optimal cutoff value of greater than 51 SBI bars corresponding to active small bowel bleeding, with sensitivity of 79.1% and specificity of 90.4%. Another study by Boal Carvalho and colleagues[48] found that in 29 patients with active bleeding, SBI had 96.6% sensitivity. Although there are promising data on the use of SBI, especially when cutoff values are applied, at this time SBI should be used only as an adjunct tool. Blue mode is another software enhancement that is a color coefficient shift of light in the short wavelength range (490–430 nm) superimposed into a white light (red, green, and blue) image, which represents computed virtual chromoendoscopy technology.[49] Blue mode imaging can improve the detection and visualization of vascular and erythematous lesions.[43,50]

Interobserver agreement

Several studies have shown high interobserver agreement with interpretation of normal and pathologic VCE findings among experts compared with trainees.[51] Petroniene and colleagues[23] showed an excellent interobserver agreement in diagnosing celiac disease among experts (kappa = 1) compared with investigators with limited VCE exposure (kappa = 0.2). Jang and colleagues[22] compared 13 experts with 10 trainees who reviewed 56 VCE video clips and found substantial agreement between experts and moderate agreement between trainees (kappa = 0.61 and kappa = 0.46, respectively). These studies highlight high interobserver agreement among experts whereas trainees need to build VCE experience in order to improve diagnostic proficiency.

Practical tips

A few practical tips from the authors when reading VCE are (1) Perform VCE read earlier in the day to avoid fatigue and lack of concentration; (2) avoid distractions because abnormalities may be visible in just a few or even in a single frame; (3) avoid reading multiple consecutive studies which can result in fatigue; (4) avoid over-interpreting clinically insignificant findings, for example, red spots; and (5) look for subtle changes, such as focal edema, clubbing of villi, and erythema, which may signal pathology.

Reporting a Video Capsule Endoscopy Examination

Standardization of VCE reporting in clinical practice has been widely recognized as a necessity. A consensus-based Capsule Endoscopy Structured Terminology (CEST) developed by a panel of experts should be utilized routinely when documenting VCE findings.[52] This allows for uniformity of reporting, optimal longitudinal patient care, assessment of quality metrics, and homogeneous data acquisition for research. The progress of embracing a universally accepted format, however, has been slow. In 2017, the American Gastroenterological Association published guidelines on elements required for appropriate and consistent documentation of VCE procedures.[19] Broadly, these components include preprocedure data, such as capsule system used, indication and type of bowel preparation, and postprocedure information, such as bowel cleanliness, relevant findings, pertinent negatives, and diagnoses.

Based on available data, the authors suggest that a VCE report should include mandatory data fields of patient identification, procedure date and reading physician, and comprehensive information, as outlined below and in **Table 3**.

Indication
The current recognized indications for VCE are small bowel bleeding, iron deficiency anemia, suspected or known Crohn disease, suspected small bowel tumors, surveillance in polyposis syndromes, evaluation of abnormal small bowel imaging, suspected or refractory celiac sprue, and other malabsorptive syndromes. The relevant *International Classification of Diseases* codes should be used when applicable for reimbursement purposes and can serve as a valuable tool for clinical trials.[52]

Landmarks and transit times
Documentation of the first gastric image, first duodenal image, and first image of the cecum allows capsule software algorithms to generate total gastric and SBTTs. The SBTT is expressed further as a percentage of the total transit time within the small bowel, which is a useful tool in determining presumptive capsule location. Rapid SBTT of less than 2 hours may lead to missed lesions.[53]

Findings
Use of CEST, as described by Korman and colleagues,[52] standardizes terminology allowing for more precise and uniform nomenclature of abnormalities, extent of changes, and other associated attributes, for example, number, size, and bleeding angioectasia. Each finding must be time stamped as hours:minutes:seconds and by percentage of SBTT. The Lewis score and Capsule Endoscopy Crohn's Disease Activity Index are well-accepted rating scales for the assessment of Crohn disease.[54–57] Other classifications, such as the Saurin classification system, have been applied,

Table 3	
Reporting a video capsule endoscopy examination	
Report	**Use Capsule Endoscopy Standard Terminology (CEST)**

Mandatory fields	1. Patient identifiers
	   a. Name
	   b. Medical record number
	   c. Date of birth
	2. Date of procedure
	3. Reading physician
	4. Capsule system used

Components	1. Indication 2. Landmarks and transit times a. Specify if incomplete examination 3. Findings 4. Images/thumbnails 5. Localization 6. Cleanliness/visualization quality 7. Diagnoses 8. Management plan

where P2 indicates a definite lesion (angiodysplastic lesion, ulceration, or neoplasm) and P1 signifies a finding of unclear certainty (red spot or erosion).[58]

Images
Captured thumbnails of identified landmarks and findings should be annotated individually and included in the report.

Localization
Determining the exact location of the capsule within the small bowel represents an area of intense clinical and research interest, particularly with the expanding role of artificial intelligence. Localization of an abnormality can be accurate at certain anatomic points, such as the ampulla or ileocecal valve. In most patients, however, localization of an image within the small bowel is relative to the SBTT. One simplistic and practical but less than precise approach is to divide SBTT into quarters representing the proximal jejunum (0%–25%), distal jejunum (26%–50%), proximal ileum (51%–75%), and distal ileum (76%–100%).[33] Based on a consensus of experts, Korman and colleagues[52] recommended dividing the SBTT into 3 equal time segments: proximal, middle, and distal small bowel. The obvious difficulty with these methods is the assumption that motility throughout the small bowel occurs at a uniform rate within the same individual. Nonetheless, attempts at estimating capsule location guide the optimal device-assisted enteroscopy approach that should be considered to reach a suspect lesion, as described by Chalazan and colleagues.[59]

Cleanliness and visualization quality
Data on the advantage of routinely prescribing a purgative bowel preparation as it relates to improved small bowel mucosal visualization remain conflicting.[33,60–62] Food residue, bubbles, and turbid fluid interfere with visualization, particularly in the distal small bowel. Irrespective of whether or not a purgative bowel preparation is administered, the VCE report should include information on the adequacy of mucosal visualization. An easy method of implementing a comprehensive scoring system for small bowel cleanliness, however, is needed. Hookey and colleagues[60] used a 5-point ordinal cleanliness scale, and Hansel and colleagues[33] used a 4-point cleanliness scale to document estimated percentage of visualized small bowel mucosa. VCE reports should record the percentage of viewable mucosa that can be ascribed to a segment of small bowel. Ultimately a VCE-based software algorithm that provides total and segmental visualization scores would be ideal and more objective.

Diagnoses
Whenever appropriate, use CEST to provide a diagnosis or overall impression, such as normal examination, angioectasia, bleeding of unknown origin, or Crohn disease.[52]

Management
A patient management plan based on VCE findings and diagnoses is an integral part of the report. The recommended strategies may include conservative follow-up versus device-assisted enteroscopy and antegrade or retrograde approaches to be specified. In patients with an incomplete small bowel examination (video capsule does not reach the cecum), recommendations to monitor for retention and perform an abdominal radiograph at 2 weeks, if passage is not witnessed, and avoiding magnetic resonance imaging should be specified. When an incomplete examination is due to delayed gastric emptying, then the option of endoscopic placement of the video capsule directly into the duodenal lumen using a dedicated delivery device should be included.

Whether a natural language or computer-generated system is used, the components of a report provide thorough and informative documentation of VCE findings and a proposed plan of management. Furthermore, more effort is required to integrate CEST into the VCE report.

SUMMARY

Structured and dedicated VCE training programs are recommended for GI trainees to master the skills of accurate capsule interpretation. Competence in performing endoscopy does not equate to competence in VCE. Direct observation of real-time cases and completing at least 25 supervised reads by a trainee are needed before competency assessment. Formalized competency assessment tools are key to overcoming the variable individual learning curves while ensuring that each trainee acquires a satisfactory level of proficiency. Online Web sites and e-learning are the future platforms for VCE training and competency evaluation, likely driven by individual GI fellowship programs or national and international GI societies. These will pave the way for training curricula of all capsule-based technology.

Interpreting a VCE examination is a time-consuming procedure that requires careful analysis of large amounts of visual data.Interpreting a VCE exam is a time-consuming procedure that requires careful analysis of large amounts of visual data which prompted the development of innovative technical software to minimize reading times and improve pathology recognition. Until robust data are available, some technology enhancements should be used as adjuncts only and not replace the need to review an entire capsule examination. The future of VCE interpretation undoubtedly will evolve to incorporate exciting advances in artificial intelligence.

A standardized format for VCE reporting that incorporates CEST should be adopted routinely into clinical practice. The components of a report provide thorough and informative documentation of VCE findings and allow for optimal patient care, assessment of quality metrics, and uniformity of data acquisition for clinical trials.

CLINICS CARE POINTS

- Structured VCE training programs and courses are beneficial for GI trainees to acquire the skills of capsule interpretation for independent practice.
- Direct observation of real-time cases and completing at least 25 supervised reads by a trainee are needed before competency assessment.
- There is high interobserver agreement with interpretation of normal and pathologic VCE findings among expert capsule endoscopists.
- A consensus-based CEST developed by a panel of experts should be utilized routinely when reporting VCE findings.

DISCLOSURE

E. Rajan: (1) Medtronic—Intellectual property; (2) Olympus—Consulting.

REFERENCES

1. Pasha SF, Leighton JA, Das A, et al. Double-balloon enteroscopy and capsule endoscopy have comparable diagnostic yield in small-bowel disease: a meta-analysis. Clin Gastroenterol Hepatol 2008;6(6):671–6.

2. Gerson LB, Fidler JL, Cave DR, et al. ACG clinical guideline: diagnosis and management of small bowel bleeding. Am J Gastroenterol 2015;110(9):1265–87 [quiz: 88].

3. Raju GS, Gerson L, Das A, et al. American Gastroenterological Association (AGA) Institute technical review on obscure gastrointestinal bleeding. Gastroenterology 2007;133(5):1697–717.

4. Gurudu SR, Bruining DH, Acosta RD, et al. The role of endoscopy in the management of suspected small-bowel bleeding. Gastrointest Endosc 2017;85(1):22–31.

5. Sabbagh R, Levi E, Antaki F. Video capsule endoscopy findings in a patient with iron deficiency anemia. Gastroenterology 2012;142(1):e12–3.

6. Carey EJ, Leighton JA, Heigh RI, et al. A single-center experience of 260 consecutive patients undergoing capsule endoscopy for obscure gastrointestinal bleeding. Am J Gastroenterol 2007;102(1):89–95.

7. Triester SL, Leighton JA, Leontiadis GI, et al. A meta-analysis of the yield of capsule endoscopy compared to other diagnostic modalities in patients with non-stricturing small bowel Crohn's disease. Am J Gastroenterol 2006;101(5):954–64.

8. Trifan A, Singeap AM, Cojocariu C, et al. Small bowel tumors in patients undergoing capsule endoscopy: a single center experience. J Gastrointest Liver Dis 2010;19(1):21–5.

9. Atlas DS, Rubio-Tapia A, Van Dyke CT, et al. Capsule endoscopy in nonresponsive celiac disease. Gastrointest Endosc 2011;74(6):1315–22.

10. Wang A, Banerjee S, Barth BA, et al. Wireless capsule endoscopy. Gastrointest Endosc 2013;78(6):805–15.

11. Gunjan D, Sharma V, Rana SS, et al. Small bowel bleeding: a comprehensive review. Gastroenterol Rep 2014;2(4):262–75.

12. Segarajasingam DS, Hanley SC, Barkun AN, et al. Randomized controlled trial comparing outcomes of video capsule endoscopy with push enteroscopy in obscure gastrointestinal bleeding. Can J Gastroenterol Hepatol 2015;29(2):85–90.

13. Teshima CW, Kuipers EJ, van Zanten SV, et al. Double balloon enteroscopy and capsule endoscopy for obscure gastrointestinal bleeding: an updated meta-analysis. J Gastroenterol Hepatol 2011;26(5):796–801.

14. Rondonotti E, Soncini M, Girelli C, et al. Small bowel capsule endoscopy in clinical practice: a multicenter 7-year survey. Eur J Gastroenterol Hepatol 2010;22(11):1380–6.

15. Koulaouzidis A, Rondonotti E, Giannakou A, et al. Diagnostic yield of small-bowel capsule endoscopy in patients with iron-deficiency anemia: a systematic review. Gastrointest Endosc 2012;76(5):983–92.

16. Faigel DO, Baron TH, Adler DG, et al. ASGE guideline: guidelines for credentialing and granting privileges for capsule endoscopy. Gastrointest Endosc 2005;61(4):503–5.

17. Rajan EA, Pais SA, Degregorio BT, et al. Small-bowel endoscopy core curriculum. Gastrointest Endosc 2013;77(1):1–6.

18. Sidhu R, Chetcuti Zammit S, Baltes P, et al. Curriculum for small-bowel capsule endoscopy and device-assisted enteroscopy training in Europe: European Society of Gastrointestinal Endoscopy (ESGE) Position Statement. Endoscopy 2020. https://doi.org/10.1055/a-1185-1289.

19. Enns RA, Hookey L, Armstrong D, et al. Clinical practice guidelines for the use of video capsule endoscopy. Gastroenterology 2017;152(3):497–514.

20. Read AJ, Rice MD, Conjeevaram HS, et al. A deeper look at the small bowel: training pathways in video capsule endoscopy and device-assisted enteroscopy. Dig Dis Sci 2018;63(9):2210–9.
21. Albert JG, Humbla O, McAlindon ME, et al. A simple evaluation tool (ET-CET) indicates increase of diagnostic skills from small bowel capsule endoscopy training courses: a prospective observational european multicenter study. Medicine 2015; 94(43):e1941.
22. Jang BI, Lee SH, Moon JS, et al. Inter-observer agreement on the interpretation of capsule endoscopy findings based on capsule endoscopy structured terminology: a multicenter study by the Korean Gut Image Study Group. Scand J Gastroenterol 2010;45(3):370–4.
23. Petroniene R, Dubcenco E, Baker JP, et al. Given capsule endoscopy in celiac disease: evaluation of diagnostic accuracy and interobserver agreement. Am J Gastroenterol 2005;100(3):685–94.
24. Sidhu R, Sakellariou P, McAlindon ME, et al. Is formal training necessary for capsule endoscopy? The largest gastroenterology trainee study with controls. Dig Liver Dis 2008;40(4):298–302.
25. Rajan E, Martinez M, Gorospe E, et al. Prospective multicenter study to evaluate capsule endoscopy competency using a validated assessment tool. Gastrointest Endosc 2020;91(5):1140–5.
26. Rajan E, Iyer PG, Oxentenko AS, et al. Training in small-bowel capsule endoscopy: assessing and defining competency. Gastrointest Endosc 2013;78(4): 617–22.
27. Postgate A, Haycock A, Thomas-Gibson S, et al. Computer-aided learning in capsule endoscopy leads to improvement in lesion recognition ability. Gastrointest Endosc 2009;70(2):310–6.
28. Velayos Jimenez B, Alcaide Suarez N, Gonzalez Redondo G, et al. Impact of the endoscopist's experience on the negative predictive value of capsule endoscopy. Gastroenterol Hepatol 2017;40(1):10–5.
29. Lim YJ, Joo YS, Jung DY, et al. Learning curve of capsule endoscopy. Clin Endosc 2013;46(6):633–6.
30. Cave DR, Fleischer DE, Leighton JA, et al. A multicenter randomized comparison of the Endocapsule and the Pillcam SB. Gastrointest Endosc 2008;68(3):487–94.
31. Koulaouzidis A, Rondonotti E, Karargyris A. Small-bowel capsule endoscopy: a ten-point contemporary review. World J Gastroenterol 2013;19(24):3726–46.
32. Westerhof J, Koornstra JJ, Hoedemaker RA, et al. Diagnostic yield of small bowel capsule endoscopy depends on the small bowel transit time. World J Gastroenterol 2012;18(13):1502–7.
33. Hansel SL, Murray JA, Alexander JA, et al. Evaluating a combined bowel preparation for small-bowel capsule endoscopy: a prospective randomized-controlled study. Gastroenterol Rep 2020;8(1):31–5.
34. Zheng Y, Hawkins L, Wolff J, et al. Detection of lesions during capsule endoscopy: physician performance is disappointing. Am J Gastroenterol 2012; 107(4):554–60.
35. Barkin JA, Barkin JS. Video Capsule Endoscopy: Technology, Reading, and Troubleshooting. Gastrointest Endosc Clin N Am 2017;27(1):15–27.
36. Günther U, Daum S, Zeitz M, et al. Capsule endoscopy: comparison of two different reading modes. Int J Colorectal Dis 2012;27(4):521–5.
37. Kyriakos N, Karagiannis S, Galanis P, et al. Evaluation of four time-saving methods of reading capsule endoscopy videos. Eur J Gastroenterol Hepatol 2012;24(11):1276–80.

38. Beg S, Wronska E, Araujo I, et al. Use of rapid reading software to reduce capsule endoscopy reading times while maintaining accuracy. Gastrointest Endosc 2020;91(6):1322-7.

39. Hosoe N, Watanabe K, Miyazaki T, et al. Evaluation of performance of the Omni mode for detecting video capsule endoscopy images: A multicenter randomized controlled trial. Endosc Int open 2016;4(8):E878-82.

40. Xu Y, Zhang W, Ye S, et al. The evaluation of the OMOM capsule endoscopy with similar pictures elimination mode. Clin Res Hepatol Gastroenterol 2014;38(6):757-62.

41. Saurin JC, Jacob P, Heyries L, et al. Multicenter prospective evaluation of the express view reading mode for small-bowel capsule endoscopy studies. Endosc Int open 2018;6(5):E616-21.

42. Gomes C, Pinho R, Ponte A, et al. Evaluation of the sensitivity of the Express View function in the Mirocam(®) capsule endoscopy software. Scand J Gastroenterol 2020;55(3):371-5.

43. Koulaouzidis A, Smirnidis A, Douglas S, et al. QuickView in small-bowel capsule endoscopy is useful in certain clinical settings, but QuickView with Blue Mode is of no additional benefit. Eur J Gastroenterol Hepatol 2012;24(9):1099-104.

44. Saurin JC, Lapalus MG, Cholet F, et al. Can we shorten the small-bowel capsule reading time with the "Quick-view" image detection system? Dig Liver Dis 2012;44(6):477-81.

45. Halling ML, Nathan T, Kjeldsen J, et al. High sensitivity of quick view capsule endoscopy for detection of small bowel Crohn's disease. J Gastroenterol Hepatol 2014;29(5):992-6.

46. Han S, Fahed J, Cave DR. Suspected Blood Indicator to Identify Active Gastrointestinal Bleeding: A Prospective Validation. Gastroenterol Res 2018;11(2):106-11.

47. Tal AO, Filmann N, Makhlin K, et al. The capsule endoscopy "suspected blood indicator" (SBI) for detection of active small bowel bleeding: no active bleeding in case of negative SBI. Scand J Gastroenterol 2014;49(9):1131-5.

48. Boal Carvalho P, Magalhães J, Dias DECF, et al. Suspected blood indicator in capsule endoscopy: a valuable tool for gastrointestinal bleeding diagnosis. Arq Gastroenterol 2017;54(1):16-20.

49. Abdelaal UM, Morita E, Nouda S, et al. Blue mode imaging may improve the detection and visualization of small-bowel lesions: A capsule endoscopy study. Saudi J Gastroenterol 2015;21(6):418-22.

50. Cotter J, Magalhães J, de Castro FD, et al. Virtual chromoendoscopy in small bowel capsule endoscopy: New light or a cast of shadow? World J Gastrointest Endosc 2014;6(8):359-65.

51. Koffas A, Laskaratos FM, Epstein O. Training in video capsule endoscopy: Current status and unmet needs. World J Gastrointest Endosc 2019;11(6):395-402.

52. Korman LY, Delvaux M, Gay G, et al. Capsule endoscopy structured terminology (CEST): proposal of a standardized and structured terminology for reporting capsule endoscopy procedures. Endoscopy 2005;37(10):951-9.

53. Buscaglia JM, Kapoor S, Clarke JO, et al. Enhanced diagnostic yield with prolonged small bowel transit time during capsule endoscopy. Int J Med Sci 2008;5(6):303-8.

54. Gralnek IM, Defranchis R, Seidman E, et al. Development of a capsule endoscopy scoring index for small bowel mucosal inflammatory change. Aliment Pharmacol Ther 2008;27(2):146-54.

55. Cotter J, Dias de Castro F, Magalhães J, et al. Validation of the Lewis score for the evaluation of small-bowel Crohn's disease activity. Endoscopy 2015;47(4):330–5.
56. Gal E, Geller A, Fraser G, et al. Assessment and validation of the new capsule endoscopy Crohn's disease activity index (CECDAI). Dig Dis Sci 2008;53(7): 1933–7.
57. Niv Y, Ilani S, Levi Z, et al. Validation of the Capsule Endoscopy Crohn's Disease Activity Index (CECDAI or Niv score): a multicenter prospective study. Endoscopy 2012;44(1):21–6.
58. Saurin JC, Delvaux M, Gaudin JL, et al. Diagnostic value of endoscopic capsule in patients with obscure digestive bleeding: blinded comparison with video push-enteroscopy. Endoscopy 2003;35(7):576–84.
59. Chalazan B, Gostout CJ, Song LM, et al. Use of Capsule Small Bowel Transit Time to Determine the Optimal Enteroscopy Approach. Gastroenterol Res 2012;5(2): 39–44.
60. Hookey L, Louw J, Wiepjes M, et al. Lack of benefit of active preparation compared with a clear fluid-only diet in small-bowel visualization for video capsule endoscopy: results of a randomized, blinded, controlled trial. Gastrointest Endosc 2017;85(1):187–93.
61. Cave DR, Hakimian S, Patel K. Current controversies concerning capsule endoscopy. Dig Dis Sci 2019;64(11):3040–7.
62. Rokkas T, Papaxoinis K, Triantafyllou K, et al. Does purgative preparation influence the diagnostic yield of small bowel video capsule endoscopy?: A meta-analysis. Am J Gastroenterol 2009;104(1):219–27.
63. Pioche M, Vanbiervliet G, Jacob P, et al. Prospective randomized comparison between axial- and lateral-viewing capsule endoscopy systems in patients with obscure digestive bleeding. Endoscopy 2014;46(6):479–84.

Preparation, Timing, Prokinetics, and Surface Agents in Video Capsule Endoscopy

Elizabeth Squirell, MD, FRCP(C)[a,1], Michelle Ricci, MD, FRCP(C)[a,1], Lawrence Hookey, MD, FRCP(C), FCAG[a,b,]*

KEYWORDS

• Video capsule endoscopy • Split dosing • Active preparation • Diagnostic yield

KEY POINTS

• There is a trend in data to support active preparation for video capsule endoscopy (VCE), but the timing of this remains unclear. Split dosing may be the most efficacious preparation.
• Study methodology continues to evolve, with increased use of standardized scales, with the addition of diagnostic yield as an outcome.
• The use of adjuncts has not been detrimental, but their value has not been proved to improve outcomes of VCE.

INTRODUCTION

The utility of purgative bowel preparation in video capsule endoscopy (VCE) has been an area of controversy since the introduction of the test in the early 2000s. Because the small bowel is much less likely to have formed stool than the colon, initial VCEs were undertaken with the expectation that bowel preparation may not be necessary for adequate visualization. Experience revealed, however, that the small bowel often has limited visibility, and some investigators have posited that bowel preparation may improve test outcomes. Incomplete tests or obscured views with inadequate visualization of the small bowel may result in missed lesions and contribute to a low diagnostic yield (DY) in VCE. Because of this, small bowel visualization quality (SBVQ), gastric transit time (GTT), and study completion rate (CR) have been incorporated along with DY as quality indicators in VCE research.[1,2]

[a] Gastrointestinal Diseases Research Unit, Department of Medicine, Queen's University, Kingston, Ontario, Canada; [b] Division of Gastroenterology, Hotel Dieu Hospital, 166 Brock Street, Kingston, Ontario K7L 5G2, Canada
[1] Co-primary authors.
* Corresponding author. Division of Gastroenterology, Hotel Dieu Hospital, 166 Brock Street, Kingston, Ontario K7L 5G2, Canada.
E-mail address: Lawrence.hookey@kingstonhsc.ca

Gastrointest Endoscopy Clin N Am 31 (2021) 251–265
https://doi.org/10.1016/j.giec.2020.12.012
1052-5157/21/© 2020 Elsevier Inc. All rights reserved.

There is good evidence in colonoscopy that a purgative bowel preparation is necessary in order to examine the colon safely and completely.[3,4] This has prompted research into the use of similar purgative bowel preparations to optimize accuracy in VCE. This article reviews the challenges in researching attempts to improve visualization, along with results of studies on whether or not to use a purgative, what timing may be best for such use, and whether adjuncts further improve results.

CHALLENGES IN STUDYING PREPARATION FOR VIDEO CAPSULE ENDOSCOPY

Research in VCE preparation has been challenged by definition of outcomes. The ideal outcome is DY, but, as is commonly the case, the numbers needed for individual trials to demonstrate differences in this often exceed feasibility. Meta-analyses have stepped in to help investigate this further.[5–7] Agreement, however, is the key issue in all of these outcomes: What is a good preparation? What is adequate? What is a positive study? and even, What value does a normal or negative study have? Preparation quality in colonoscopy and subsequently VCE has been assessed by scales, ranging from inadequate to excellent, with variation in-between. Although colonoscopy research now has excellent validated quality control tools for bowel preparation, VCE research is making progress but continues to explore options.[8] The authors previously have used a qualitative scale, with each examination assessed by 3 reviewers, preceded by a pretrial agreement exercise, and assessment for agreement at the end of the trial.[9] Van Weyenberg and colleagues[10] reported, however, a computerized assessment of cleanliness tool, using the color bars on the VCE display. This correlated well with qualitative scale results.

How to define DY is another methodological challenge for VCE research. First, the examination may find something, but was it related to the indication, or is it an incidental finding? If the result is the latter, is the study still diagnostic? Some studies consider any finding diagnostic and others look for sources of bleeding in those indications, whereas others use other criteria.[1,11–14]

PURGATIVE OR NO?

As summarized in **Tables 1** and **2**, there have been 3 meta-analyses of randomized controlled trials (RCTs) undertaken comparing purgative bowel preparation to fasting or clear fluids. The earliest of these, in a 2012 study by Belsey and colleagues,[7] found a higher DY in those using polyethylene glycol (PEG)–electrolyte lavage solution (ELS) preparation before VCE and no benefit to sodium phosphate (NaP) preparation. Similarly, a 2014 meta-analysis of 10 RCTs by Kotwal and colleagues[6] concluded that a purgative bowel preparation could improve SBVQ with variable effects on DY. In 2017, Wu and colleagues[5] conducted a meta-analysis that included only PEG-based bowel preparation compared with fasting or clear fluids. This study also concluded that PEG-based bowel preparation likely improved SBVQ and DY, but further rigorous RCTs were required.

At the time of these meta-analyses, there were no high-powered RCTs available on the subject and the available literature was limited to small studies with significant variability in the control and intervention groups. There was significant heterogeneity demonstrated in 2 of the 3 meta-analyses, and studies included were limited by lack of standardization in SBVQ measurement as well as variability in control groups. This literature may support the use of purgative bowel preparations for VCE, but the need for high-powered, rigorous RCTs was demonstrated by each meta-analysis.[5–7]

Postgate and colleagues[15] undertook a large RCT in 2009 that compared purgative bowel preparation (magnesium citrate, with or without a motility agent) to clear fluids.

Table 1
Timing of bowel preparation

Authors	Sample Size	Experiment	Control	Findings	Conclusion
Wu et al,[16] 2020	70/72/70/72/70	Group B: 1-L PEG-ELS 12 h before VCE Group C: 2-L PEG-ELS 12 h before VCE Group D: 1-L PEG-ELS 4 h before VCE Group E: 2-L PEG-ELS 4 h before VCE	Group A: 12 h fast	Group D had significantly better SBVQ than A (66.3% vs 32.5%; P = <0.001) DY was higher in groups C, D, and E	1 L of PEG-ELS 4 h prior to VCE is superior in cleansing the small bowel, with better tolerance than a 2-L preparation.
Magalhães-Costa et al,[20] 2016	29/28	1-L PEG-ELS at 2000 1-L PEG-ELS at 0900 VCE at 1400	2-L PEG-ELS at 2000 VCE at 0900	No significant difference in DY Difference in extent of mucosa visualized (P = .045) and fluid/ debris ratio (P = .016) favoring split preparation	Split-dose regimen improved mucosal visualization with no difference in DY
Black et al,[21] 2015	17/17	2-L PEG-ELS 4 h prior to VCE	2-L PEG-ELS 14 h prior to VCE	No significant difference in SBVQ between groups (P = .091) Similar DY between groups (53% vs 47%; P = 1.00)	The difference between day before and same-day bowel preparation is not significant.

Table 2
Use of purgative bowel preparation

	Consensus Guidelines	
Authors	Recommendation and Rationale	Level of Recommendation
European Rondonotti et al,[18] 2018	Purgative bowel preparation with 2-L PEG-ELS prior to VCE Based on multiple meta-analyses that have identified bowel preparation as useful in improving SBVQ. Timing of bowel preparation is felt to be unclear at this point.	Strong, high-quality evidence
Canadian Enns et al,[17] 2017	Purgative bowel preparation before VCE Based on meta-analyses that have identified improved visualization quality. The consensus group did not find convincing evidence to recommend between NaP and PEG-ELS preparation.	Strong, low-quality evidence

	Meta-analysis		
Authors	Studies Included	Findings	Limitations	Conclusion
Wu et al,[5] 2017	9 RCTs PEG-ELS vs clear fluid	PEG-ELS—improved SBVQ and DY. No difference in CR	Blinding unclear in some included studies Variability in control group Small sample sizes of included studies No uniform reporting of SBVQ	PEG-based bowel preparation has improved DY and SBVQ. Further study is needed.

Authors	Sample Size	Purgative	Control	Findings	Conclusion
Kotwal et al,[6] 2014	7 RCTs (purgative vs clear fluid) 3 RCTs (purgative + antifoaming agent vs clear fluid)		NaP—no benefit over control P/MC—improved DY, no difference in SBVQ PEG-ELS—improved DY and SBVQ	Significant heterogeneity Variability in control group Small sample sizes of included studies	It is possible that bowel purgatives improved DY and SBVQ, but further rigorous RCTs are required.
Belsey et al,[7] 2012	8 RCTs		PEG-ELS—improved DY NaP—no benefit over control	Significant heterogeneity Variability in control group Small sample sizes of included studies No uniform reporting of SBVQ	PEG-based bowel preparation has improved DY, but NaP does not.
Randomized Controlled Trials (Not Included in Above Meta-analyses)					
Authors	Sample Size	Purgative	Control	Findings	Conclusion
Wu et al,[16] 2020	70/72/70/72/70	Group B: 1-L PEG-ELS 12 h before VCE Group C: 2-L PEG-ELS 12 h before VCE Group D: 1-L PEG-ELS 4 h before VCE Group E: 2-L PEG-ELS 4 h before VCE	Group A: 12 h fast	Group D had significantly better SBVQ than A (66.3% vs 32.5%; $P = <0.001$) DY was higher in group C, D, and E	1L of PEG-ELS 4 h prior to VCE is superior in cleansing the small bowel with better tolerance than a 2-L preparation.s
Hookey et al,[9] 2017	63/60/59	2 sachets P/MC or 2-L PEG-ELS qhs before VCE	Clear fluids only the evening before	No difference on DY or SBVQ (5-point ordinal score or computerized score) Improved tolerability of clear fluid preparation	No significant benefit of purgative bowel preparations compared with clear fluids prior to VCE.
Postgate et al,[15] 2009	40/37/38	Senna + Citramag Or Senna + Citramag + Maxeran	Clear fluids + 10 h fast	No difference in DY after correction for multiple testing of data No difference CR, GTT	No significant benefit of bowel purgatives over standard preparation in reducing GTT or CR or view quality.

Despite its large sample size (150 participants randomized) and early publication, the concomitant study of motility agents led to a study design that could not be incorporated into any of the previously discussed meta-analyses. Their study found no significant difference in their primary outcomes of GTT, SBVQ, or CR or their secondary outcome of DY.[15]

The 2 largest RCTs on this topic were published later than, and therefore not included in, the meta-analyses, discussed previously. Hookey and colleagues[9] (2017) found that purgative bowel preparation had no benefit over clear fluids alone in SBVQ or DY. This study included 198 randomized participants and used a computerized scoring system for visualization quality in order to assist in standardizing future research on SBVQ.[9] Both Hookey and colleagues[9] and Postgate and colleagues[15] found that clear fluid preparation was tolerated significantly better than purgative bowel preparation.

In 2019, Wu and colleagues[16] undertook the largest RCT on the topic, with 410 randomized participants. They compared PEG-ELS preparation (2 L or 1 L at 12 hours or 4 hours prior to VCE) to 12 hours of fasting. This study found significant improvement in SBVQ in those who underwent 1-L PEG-ELS preparation 4 hours prior to VCE compared with controls.[16]

ASSOCIATION GUIDELINES

A 2017 Canadian guideline and a 2018 European technical review of their 2015 guideline make recommendations on bowel preparation in VCE. Although they both recognize that further research is warranted, specifically into the timing of preparation administration, they make strong recommendations to administer a purgative bowel preparation prior to VCE. These recommendations are based primarily on the meta-analyses, discussed previously.[17–19]

TIMING OF PURGATIVES

At this point in time, the majority of literature on the use of a purgative bowel preparation involves preparation 12 hours prior to VCE.[5–7] Unfortunately, SBVQ is limited across studies regardless of preparation choice. Bowel preparation in colonoscopy has been shown to have higher yield when taken in split dosing, with the last dose taken approximately 4 hours prior to examination. Physiologically, it then may be logical that the small bowel would have optimal visualization with preparation taken at a similar or shorter interval than that of a colonoscopy. Three recent RCTs using PEG-based bowel preparations have attempted to address this question with various approaches.[16,20,21]

In 2015, Black and colleagues[21] compared 2 L of PEG-ELS taken either 14 hours or 4 hours prior to VCE. This was a low-powered, small study, with only 34 participants randomized. They found that there was no difference in SBVQ or DY between groups.[21] Similarly, Magalhães-Costa and colleagues (2016) randomized patients to 1 L of PEG-ELS in the evening and 1 L of PEG-ELS in the morning or 2-L PEG-ELS in the evening before VCE. This study found that split-dose PEG-ELS improves the extent of the mucosa visualized but not the DY. This study also was limited in power by the small number of randomized participants (n = 57).[20]

Finally, a rigorous 2019 study reviewed the use of PEG-ELS in 1 L or 2 L either 12 hours or 4 hours prior to VCE. They compared each group to a control group who underwent a 12-hour fast prior to VCE. Overall, there was a significantly better SBVQ in patients who underwent 1-L PEG-ELS preparation 4 hours prior to VCE. There was increased turbidity of fluid seen in the larger-volume (2-L) group, which may play a role in the negative results of many of the previous studies.[16]

CHOICE OF BOWEL PREPARATION

Kotwal and colleagues[6] suggest that PEG bowel preparations may improve both DY and SBVQ, whereas sodium picosulfate plus magnesium citrate (P/MC) may improve DY but not SBVQ, and NaP preparation does not lead to improvement in either. In contrast, in a 2009 meta-analysis that included retrospective studies, Rokkas and colleagues[22] performed a subgroup analysis that suggested P/MC may lead to higher SBVQ than PEG preparation. Given the borderline significance ($P = .046$ for P/MC and $P = .062$ for PEG), further study was suggested. The European Society of Gastrointestinal Endoscopy guidelines suggest the use of 2 L of PEG over other purgative choices, whereas the Canadian guidelines do not make a recommendation on choice of preparation.[17–19]

Again, more research into choice and timing of bowel preparation appears necessary. The use of NaP preparation has been withdrawn from the North American market due to an elevated risk of adverse effects (ie, acute kidney injury) and has negligible supporting evidence.[23] Thus, it is not recommended. There is limited evidence that may favor PEG preparation over P/MC, but further research is warranted.[6,17,18,22]

ADJUNCTS AND SURFACE AGENTS

Mucosal visualization, DY, and completion of the capsule to the level of the cecum before the battery dies are affected by air bubbles, food material/bile in the bowel, and delayed GTT and intestinal transit time. There have been multiple studies performed to look at adjunctive therapy in addition to purgatives to address these issues in the hope of improving visualization, CRs, and DY.

Prokinetic Agents

In the early days of VCE, the battery life was 8 hours, and up to 20% of video capsules did not complete transit through the small bowel before the end of the battery life.[24] Modern capsules have an extended battery life of up to 12 hours and consequently CRs have improved to approximately 90%.[25] In theory, the use of prokinetics in bowel preparation may shorten GTT and small bowel transit time, thereby improving CRs. The caveat to decreasing transit time of the capsule, in particular, small bowel transit time, however, is that it may come at the expense of DY, if the capsule transit is too rapid to allow to acceptable mucosal visualization. To date, the use of erythromycin, metoclopramide, domperidone, lubiprostone, and prucalopride in VCE preparation has been studied with varying degrees of purgatives and multiple different study designs.[15,26–32] The results are summarized in **Table 3**. Although 3 studies show improvement in GTT,[28,30,31] 1 study shows improvement in each small bowel transit time[29] and CR[31]; overall, there is no improvement in DY.[22] Given that VCE is a diagnostic test, this raises the question if prokinetic agents have any utility as adjuncts in bowel preparation for VCE. No studies have addressed different patient populations (ie, those with gastroparesis or other slow-transit disorders), so it remains unknown if prokinetic agents may be useful in this patient population.

Simethicone

Simethicone is used in endoscopy to reduce the volume of small bubbles in the bowel lumen, because they can limit visualization. It reduces surface tension on bubbles, causing small bubbles to coalesce, thereby improving mucosal visualization. Trials consistently have shown better visualization quality in both proximal and distal small bowel with simethicone due to reduction of air bubbles; however, there are mixed results in terms of the impact of simethicone on small bowel transit time.[33–38] The use of

Table 3
Summary of studies from 2008–2020 on the use of adjuncts in video capsule enteroscopy bowel preparation

	Study Design	Intervention	Comparison	Participants	Outcome
Prokinetics					
Postgate et al,[15] 2009	Single-center Single-blind RCT	CSM: Citramag + senna + 10-mg metoclopramide	S: npo and simethicone at VCE; M: standard + 10-mg metoclopramide; CS: Citramag and senna	150 (S = 37; M = 37; CS = 39; CSM = 37)	GGT: Y, NSD SBTT: Y, NSD SBVQ: Y, NSD DY: Y, NSD CR: Y, NSD
Westerhof et al,[31] 2014	Single-center Prospective cohort study	Erythromycin, 250 mg, 1 h prior to VCE + PEG (3 L)	Domperidone, 10 mg, immediately prior to VCE + PEG (3 L)	648 (intervention 239; comparison 410)	GTT: Y, intervention; $P = .03$ SBTT: Y, NSD SBVQ: N DY: Y, NSD CR: Y, intervention; $P<.001$
Niv et al,[27] 2008	Two-center Retrospective blinded review	200-mg po erythromycin 1 h prior to VCE	12-h fast	100 (intervention 50; comparison 50)	GGT: Y, NSD SBTT: Y, NSD SBVQ: Y, NSD DY: N CR: N
Matsuura et al,[32] 2017	Single-center Double-blind, placebo-control, 2-way crossover study	24-µg lubiprostone 120 min prior to VCE	Placebo 120 min prior to VCE	20	GTT: Y, NSD SBTT: Y, NSD SBVQ: Y, intervention; $P<.001$ DY: N CR: N
Hooks et al,[28] 2009	Single-center Double-blind, placebo-controlled trial	24-µg lubiprostone 30 min prior to VCE	Placebo 30 min prior to VCE	40 (intervention 20; comparison 20)	GTT: Y, intervention; $P = .0095$ SBTT: Y, NSD SBVQ: Y, NSD DY: N CR: N

Study	Design	Intervention	Comparison	Sample size	Outcomes
McFarlane et al,[30] 2018	Single-center Retrospective chart review	Domperidone, 20 mg, prior to VCE	No domperidone prior to VCE	63 (intervention 31; comparison 33)	GTT: Y, comparison; $P = .01$ SBTT: Y, NSD SBVQ: N DY: Y, no statistical analysis CR: N
Almeida et al,[26] 2010	Single-center Randomized, single-blind RCT	10-mg metoclopramide 15 min prior to VCE	No metoclopramide	95 (intervention 47; comparison 48)	GTT: Y, NSD SBTT: Y, NSD SBVQ: Y, NSD DY: Y, NSD CR: Y, NSD
Alsahafi et al,[29] 2017	Single-center Case series	Prucalopride, 2 mg, + PEG (2 L)	PEG (2 L)	54 (intervention 29; comparison 25)	GTT: Y, NSD SBTT: Y, intervention; $P<.001$ SBVQ: N DY: N CR: Y, NSD
Simethicone					
Wei et al,[33] 2008	Single-center Randomized trial	PS: simethicone, 300 mg, 20 min prior to VCE plus PEG (1 L)	P: PEG alone (1 L) C: clear fluids alone	90 (PS 30; P 30; C 30)	GTT: Y, NSD SBTT: N SBVQ: Y, PS > P and C; $P = .001$ DY: N CR: Y, NSD
Chen et al,[34] 2011	Single-center Randomized trial	D: C + 20 mL simethicone 20 min prior to VCE	A: clear fluids B: 250-mL 20% mannitol at 5:00 d of VCE C: B + 250 mL 20% mannitol 20:00 night before VCE	193 (A 47; B 49; C 48; D 49)	GTT: Y, NSD SBTT: Y, NSD SBVQ: Y, A > C and A > D; $P = .001$ DY: Y, C and D > A and B; $P = .005$ CR: N

(continued on next page)

Table 3
(continued)

	Study Design	Intervention	Comparison	Participants	Outcome
Krijbolder et al,[35] 2018	Single-center Retrospective, Single-blind Cohort study	Simethicone (82.4 mg prior to VCE) + PEG (2 L)	PEG (2 L)	57 (intervention 27; comparison 30)	GTT: N SBTT: Y, NSD SBVQ: Y; intervention; *P*<.001 DY: Y, NSD CR: N
Papamichael et al,[36] 2015	Single-center Observational, prospective	Simethicone, 80 mg, 12 h and 1 h prior to VCE and PEG (2 L)	PEG (2 L)	114 (intervention 56; comparison 58)	GTT: Y, NSD SBTT: Y, NSD SBVQ: Y, intervention in proximal bowel; *P* = .032 DY: Y, NSD CR: Y, NSD
Esaki et al,[37] 2009	Single-center Retrospective case series	Simethicone, 200 mg, 30 min prior to VCE	Magnesium citrate 34 g, 3 h prior to VCE	75 (intervention 39, comparison 36)	GTT: Y, NSD SBTT: Y, NSD SBVQ: Y, NSD DY: Y, comparison; *P*<.01 CR: N
Fang et al,[38] 2009	Single-center RCT	Simethicone, 600 mg, 20 min prior to VCE and PEG (2 L)	PEG alone (2 L)	64 (intervention 32; comparison 32)	GTT: Y, NSD SBTT: Y, intervention; *P* = .003 SBVQ: Y, intervention; *P*<.001 DY: N CR: N
Spada et al,[40] 2010	Single-center RCT	Simethicone and PEG 16 h prior to VCE	Clear fluids day before	58 (intervention 29, comparison 29)	GTT: Y, NSD SBTT: Y, NSD SBVQ: Y, NSD DY: Y, NSD CR: Y, NSD

Rosa et al,[39] 2013	Single-center RCT	C: B + Simethicone, 100 mg, 30 min before VCE	A: fasting + 24-h liquid B: A+ 2-L PEG	57 (A 20, B 19, C 20)	GTT: Y, NSD SBTT: Y, NSD SBVQ: Y, NSD DY: Y, NSD CR: Y, NSD
Other adjuncts					
Kim et al,[41] 2014	Single-center Single-blind case control	Coffee enema with split 2-L PEG	2-L PEG preparation	34 (intervention 17; comparison 17)	GTT: Y, NSD SBTT: Y, NSD SBVQ: Y, intervention no statistical analysis DY: Y, NSD CR: N
Ou et al,[43] 2014	Single-center Single-blind RCT	Chewing gum 20 min/2 h from capsule ingestion + standard bowel preparation (2-L PEG)	Standard bowel preparation alone (2-L PEG)	122 (intervention 60; comparison 62)	GTT: Y, NSD SBTT: Y, NSD SBVQ: N DY: Y, NSD CR: Y, NSD
Apostolopoulos et al,[42] 2008	Single-center Single-blind RCT	Chewing gum 30 min/2 h from capsule ingestion + NaP	NaP	93 (intervention 47, comparison 46)	GTT: Y, intervention; $P = .045$ SBTT: Y, intervention; $P = .032$ SBVQ: Y, NSD DY: N CR: Y, NSD

Abbreviations: CF, clear fluid; N, no; NSD, no significant difference; SBTT, small bowel transit time; Y, yes.

simethicone as an adjunct does not appear to have any significant effect on DY in studies that addressed this.[33–40]

Other Adjuncts

Coffee stimulates peristalsis and helps flush bile through the gastrointestinal (GI) tract. It also stimulates, however, the release of bile via dilation of biliary ducts. Timing of administration must be done in a way that it limits excess bile release but facilitates the movement of bile, because bile is a factor that limits mucosal views. A 2014 case-control study did not note a difference in transit time; however, it suggested improved visualization in the mid–small bowel, distal small bowel, and terminal ileum when a coffee enema is administered between PEG doses with a split PEG regimen, with no effect on DY. There were 16 individuals each in the treatment and control groups for this study, and, with low participant numbers, it is not possible to make any recommendations regarding the role of coffee enemas in bowel preparation for VCE. Furthermore, the timing of the enema between the split dosing of PEG may be onerous on the patient and unnecessarily complicate the instructions for the bowel preparation for no proved clinical benefit and perhaps even to the detriment of the DY if the bowel preparation instructions became too complex for a typical patient to follow.[41]

Sugarless chewing gum is used routinely after colorectal surgery. Surgical literature has shown chewing gum to be effective in reducing ileus and promoting gut motility in the postoperative period. There are several potential mechanisms in which sugarless chewing gum may help promote GI tract motility, including (1) mimicking feeding and inducing cholinergic stimulation of the GI tract, (2) increasing salivary flow and gastric secretions, and (3) having an osmotic effect via artificial sweetener. There are 2 RCTs that have examined the effect of sugarless chewing gum on VCE bowel preparation, with 1 showing a statistically significant improvement in GTT and small bowel transit time, and 1 showing no statistically significant difference in transit time. Both studies had similar protocol with respect to chewing gum intervention but were different in the bowel purgative used prior to VCE, which raises the question if this difference is due to chewing gum or to selection of purgative. Regardless, both studies agree that visualization quality, DY, and CR do not show a significant improvement if chewing gum is administered, suggesting that sugarless chewing gum does not provide a diagnostically meaningful benefit to VCE.[42,43]

The use of adjuncts in VCE bowel preparation remains questionable. The available studies are heterogeneous in terms of interventions (dosing and timing of adjunct administration) and bowel preparations (PEG-based vs clear fluids/fasting and volumes of PEG used), making it difficult to compare 1 study to another. This lack of standardization in bowel preparation used in these studies may help explain the variability of outcomes seen even among the same adjunctive interventions. Furthermore, the sample sizes in the studies are small. This, combined with variability/heterogeneity, means that meta-analyses are unlikely to provide any further clarity for recommendation of the use of adjuncts in small bowel preparation in VCE. The current literature does not support the use of adjunctive agents in VCE bowel preparation on a routine basis.

SUMMARY

As reviewed in this article, when it comes to VCE, most questions remain unanswered: whether to use a preparation, when to use one, which particular one to use, and if anything adding along with a preparation helps, Although efforts have been made to address these questions, a more concerted effort, with further multicenter randomized factorial trials, could answer them definitively and define the standard of care. We are left with using best available literature and expert consensus.

CLINICS CARE POINTS

- Current North American and European guidelines make "strong" recommendations to administer PEG based on meta-nalyses that were done prior to the availability of the existence of RCTs, and 2/3 RCTs do not show the superiority of PEG over clear fluids and fasting, which does draw into the question a "strong recommendation".
- There is fairly significant heterogeneity in the bowel preparations used, so it is difficult to say what the "best" way to prepare the bowel is in terms of administration of prep and timing.
- It is difficult to determine if adjuvant therapies are beneficial/play an important role until there is a more standardized prep used - the studies that exist use many different bowel preparations in conjunction with the adjunctive agents so comparing one study to another and making any firm conclusions on their use is really not possible.

REFERENCES

1. Kharazmi AA, Aslani S, Kristiansen MF, et al. Indications and diagnostic yield of small-bowel capsule endoscopy in a real-world setting. BMC Gastroenterol 2020; 20. https://doi.org/10.1186/s12876-020-01326-8.
2. Grigg-Gutierrez N, Laboy C, Ramos L, et al. Diagnostic yield of video capsule endoscopy for small bowel bleeding: eight consecutive years of experience at the VA Caribbean Healthcare System. P R Health Sci J 2016;35(2):93–6.
3. Enestvedt BK, Tofani C, Laine LA, et al. 4-Liter split-dose polyethylene glycol is superior to other bowel preparations, based on systematic review and meta-analysis. Clin Gastroenterol Hepatol 2012;10(11):1225–31.
4. Gurudu SR, Ramirez FC, Harrison ME, et al. Increased adenoma detection rate with system-wide implementation of a split-dose preparation for colonoscopy. Gastrointest Endosc 2012;76(3):603–8.e1.
5. Wu S, Gao Y-J, Ge Z-Z. Optimal use of polyethylene glycol for preparation of small bowel video capsule endoscopy: a network meta-analysis. Curr Med Res Opin 2017;33(6):1149–54.
6. Kotwal VS, Attar BM, Gupta S, et al. Should bowel preparation, antifoaming agents, or prokinetics be used before video capsule endoscopy? A systematic review and meta-analysis. Eur J Gastroenterol Hepatol 2014;26(2):137–45.
7. Belsey J, Crosta C, Epstein O, et al. Meta-analysis: efficacy of small bowel preparation for small bowel video capsule endoscopy. Curr Med Res Opin 2012; 28(12):1883–90.
8. Brotz C, Nandi N, Conn M, et al. A validation study of 3 grading systems to evaluate small-bowel cleansing for wireless capsule endoscopy: a quantitative index, a qualitative evaluation, and an overall adequacy assessment. Gastrointest Endosc 2009;69(2):262–70.e1.
9. Hookey L, Louw J, Wiepjes M, et al. Lack of benefit of active preparation compared with a clear fluid–only diet in small-bowel visualization for video capsule endoscopy: results of a randomized, blinded, controlled trial. Gastrointest Endosc 2017;85(1):187–93.

10. Van Weyenberg S, De Leest H, Mulder C. Description of a novel grading system to assess the quality of bowel preparation in video capsule endoscopy. Endoscopy 2011;43(05):406–11.

11. Ben-Soussan E, Savoye G, Antonietti M, et al. Is a 2-Liter PEG preparation useful before capsule endoscopy? J Clin Gastroenterol 2005;39(5):381–4.

12. Viazis N, Sgouros S, Papaxoinis K, et al. Bowel preparation increases the diagnostic yield of capsule endoscopy: a prospective, randomized, controlled study. Gastrointest Endosc 2004;60(4):534–8.

13. van Tuyl SaC, den Ouden H, Stolk MFJ, et al. Optimal preparation for video capsule endoscopy: a prospective, randomized, single-blind study. Endoscopy 2007;39(12):1037–40.

14. Costamagna G, Shah SK, Riccioni ME, et al. A prospective trial comparing small bowel radiographs and video capsule endoscopy for suspected small bowel disease. Gastroenterology 2002;123(4):999–1005.

15. Postgate A, Tekkis P, Patterson N, et al. Are bowel purgatives and prokinetics useful for small-bowel capsule endoscopy? A prospective randomized controlled study. Gastrointest Endosc 2009;69(6):1120–8.

16. Wu S, Zhong L, Zheng P, et al. Low-dose and same day use of polyethylene glycol improves image of video capsule endoscopy: A multi-center randomized clinical trial. J Gastroenterol Hepatol 2020;35(4):634–40.

17. Enns RA, Hookey L, Armstrong D, et al. Clinical Practice Guidelines for the Use of Video Capsule Endoscopy. Gastroenterology 2017;152(3):497–514.

18. Rondonotti E, Spada C, Adler S, et al. Small-bowel capsule endoscopy and device-assisted enteroscopy for diagnosis and treatment of small-bowel disorders: European Society of Gastrointestinal Endoscopy (ESGE) Technical Review. Endoscopy 2018;50(04):423–46.

19. Pennazio M, Spada C, Eliakim R, et al. Small-bowel capsule endoscopy and device-assisted enteroscopy for diagnosis and treatment of small-bowel disorders: European Society of Gastrointestinal Endoscopy (ESGE) Clinical Guideline. Endoscopy 2015;47(04):352–86.

20. Magalhães-Costa P, Carmo J, Bispo M, et al. Superiority of the Split-dose PEG Regimen for Small-Bowel Capsule Endoscopy: A Randomized Controlled Trial. J Clin Gastroenterol 2016;50(7):e65–70.

21. Black KR, Truss W, Joiner CI, et al. A Single-Center Randomized Controlled Trial Evaluating Timing of Preparation for Capsule Enteroscopy. Clin Endosc 2015; 48(3):234.

22. Rokkas T, Papaxoinis K, Triantafyllou K, et al. Does purgative preparation influence the diagnostic yield of small bowel video capsule endoscopy?: a meta-analysis. Am J Gastroenterol 2009;104(1):219–27.

23. Rex DK, Vanner SJ. Colon cleansing before colonoscopy: Does oral sodium phosphate solution still make sense? Can J Gastroenterol 2009;23(3):210.

24. Wang A, Banerjee S, Barth BA, et al. Wireless capsule endoscopy. Gastrointest Endosc 2013;78(6):805–15.

25. Robertson KD, Singh R. Capsule endoscopy. StatPearls Publishing; 2020. Available at: https://www.ncbi.nlm.nih.gov/books/NBK482306/. Accessed December 2, 2020.

26. Almeida N, Figueiredo P, Freire P, et al. The effect of metoclopramide in capsule enteroscopy. Dig Dis Sci 2010;55(1):153.

27. Niv E, Bogner I, Barkay O, et al. Effect of erythromycin on image quality and transit time of capsule endoscopy: A two-center study. World J Gastroenterol 2008;14(16):2561.

28. Hooks SB, Rutland TJ, Di Palma JA. Lubiprostone neither decreases gastric and small-bowel transit time nor improves visualization of small bowel for capsule endoscopy: a double-blind, placebo-controlled study. Gastrointest Endosc 2009;70(5):942–6.

29. Alsahafi M, Cramer P, Chatur N, et al. The Effect of Prucalopride on Small Bowel Transit Time in Hospitalized Patients Undergoing Capsule Endoscopy. Can J Gastroenterol Hepatol 2017;2017. https://doi.org/10.1155/2017/2696947.

30. Mcfarlane M, Liu B, Nwokolo C. Domperidone prolongs oral to duodenal transit time in video capsule endoscopy. Eur J Clin Pharmacol 2018;74(4):521–4.

31. Westerhof J, Weersma RK, Hoedemaker RA, et al. Completion rate of small bowel capsule endoscopy is higher after erythromycin compared to domperidone. BMC Gastroenterol 2014;14(1):162.

32. Matsuura M, Inamori M, Inou Y, et al. Lubiprostone improves visualization of small bowel for capsule endoscopy: a double-blind, placebo-controlled 2-way cross-over study. Endosc Int Open 2017;5(6):E424.

33. Wei W, Ge Z-Z, Lu H, et al. Purgative bowel cleansing combined with simethicone improves capsule endoscopy imaging. Am J Gastroenterol 2008;103(1):77–82.

34. Chen H, Huang Y, Chen S, et al. Small bowel preparations for capsule endoscopy with mannitol and simethicone: a prospective, randomized, clinical trial. J Clin Gastroenterol 2011. https://doi.org/10.1097/MCG.0b013e3181f0f3a3.

35. Krijbolder M, Grooteman K, Bogers S, et al. Addition of simethicone improves small bowel capsule endoscopy visualisation quality. The Netherlands journal of medicine. 2018. Available at: https://pubmed.ncbi.nlm.nih.gov/29380729/. Accessed December 2, 2020.

36. Papamichael K, Karatzas P, Theodoropoulos I, et al. Simethicone adjunct to polyethylene glycol improves small bowel capsule endoscopy imaging in non-Crohn's disease patients. Ann Gastroenterol 2015. Available at: https://pubmed.ncbi.nlm.nih.gov/26423317/. Accessed December 2, 2020.

37. Esaki M, Matsumoto T, Kudo T, et al. Bowel preparations for capsule endoscopy: a comparison between simethicone and magnesium citrate. Gastrointest Endosc 2009. https://doi.org/10.1016/j.gie.2008.04.054.

38. Fang Y, Chen C, Zhang B. Effect of small bowel preparation with simethicone on capsule endoscopy. J Zhejiang Univ Sci B 2009;10(1):46–51.

39. Rosa BJF. Oral purgative and simethicone before small bowel capsule endoscopy. World J Gastrointest Endosc 2013;5(2):67.

40. Spada C, Riccioni ME, Familiari P, et al. Polyethylene glycol plus simethicone in small-bowel preparation for capsule endoscopy. Dig Liver Dis 2010;42(5):365–70.

41. Kim ES, Chun HJ, Keum B, et al. Coffee enema for preparation for small bowel video capsule endoscopy: a pilot study. Clin Nutr Res 2014;3(2):134.

42. Apostolopoulos P, Kalantzis C, Gralnek IM, et al. Clinical trial: effectiveness of chewing-gum in accelerating capsule endoscopy transit time - a prospective randomized, controlled pilot study. Aliment Pharmacol Ther 2008;28(4):405–11.

43. Ou G, Svarta S, Chan C, et al. The effect of chewing gum on small-bowel transit time in capsule endoscopy: a prospective, randomized trial. Gastrointest Endosc 2014;79(4):630–6.

Indications, Contraindications, and Considerations for Video Capsule Endoscopy

Jacquelyn G. Bolwell, MD[a], Daniel Wild, MD[b],*

KEYWORDS

- Video capsule endoscopy • Indications • Contraindications

KEY POINTS

- Video capsule endoscopy has a broad range of indications including evaluation of gastrointestinal bleeding, suspected and established Crohn's disease, refractory celiac disease and polyposis syndromes.
- The only absolute contraindication to video capsule endoscopy is luminal gastrointestinal tract obstruction; other considerations include the possibility of incomplete examination, missed lesions, and capsule retention.
- Video capsule endoscopy can be performed safely in patients with implantable cardiac devices, including pacemakers.

INTRODUCTION

Video capsule endoscopy (VCE) allows for direct visualization of the entire length of the small intestine, making it an ideal modality to evaluate a wide spectrum of disorders, including gastrointestinal (GI) bleeding, Crohn's disease, celiac disease, and polyposis syndromes (**Table 1**). This article provides the current evidence and a discussion on the indications for and contraindications to using VCE in clinical practice.

INDICATIONS FOR VIDEO CAPSULE ENDOSCOPY
Gastrointestinal Bleeding

It is estimated that approximately 5% of all GI bleeding arises from the small bowel, in areas not seen with conventional upper endoscopy and colonoscopy.[1] Bleeding from the small bowel can be indolent, presenting as iron deficiency anemia, or overt, with

a Duke University Medical Center, 1151 Duke South, Yellow Zone, Box 3534, Durham, NC 27710, USA; b Division of Gastroenterology, Duke University Medical Center, Durham, NC, USA
* Corresponding author. 302 Parkridge Avenue, Chapel Hill, NC 27517.
E-mail address: daniel.wild@duke.edu

Gastrointest Endoscopy Clin N Am 31 (2021) 267–276
https://doi.org/10.1016/j.giec.2020.12.002
1052-5157/21/© 2020 Elsevier Inc. All rights reserved.

Table 1	
Indication, contraindications and considerations for performing VCE	
Indications	**Contraindications**
Suspected GI bleeding	Luminal GI tract obstruction
Suspected Crohn's disease	*Considerations*
Monitoring known Crohn's disease	Incomplete examination
Evaluation of refractory symptoms in celiac disease	Capsule retention
Polyposis syndromes (FAP, Peutz–Jeghers syndrome)	Missed lesion
	Implantable cardiac devices

melena or even hematochezia and hemodynamic compromise. VCE has a role in both of these settings.[2]

In the absence of hematemesis, VCE is indicated as the next step to investigate overt GI bleeding if high-quality EGD and colonoscopy are nondiagnostic.[3] When performed in this context, a meta-analysis of 10 studies found its pooled diagnostic yield to be 62%.[4] Positive findings are more likely on VCE when bleeding is overt, a patient's hemoglobin level is less than 10 g/dL or has decreased by more than 4 g/dL.[3,5] Randomized controlled data show that VCE is superior to both conventional small bowel radiography and angiography for the evaluation of overt bleeding suspected to arise from small bowel bleeding with diagnostic yields of 30% versus 7% compared with conventional radiography and 53.3% versus 20% compared with angiography.[6,7] VCE has also been shown to be superior to push enteroscopy in evaluating patients with suspected small bowel bleeding, with diagnostic yields of 72.5% versus 48.7%.[8]

When performed for suspected overt small bowel bleeding, VCE should be performed as close to the bleeding event as possible, because this practice increases its diagnostic yield.[3] A large retrospective study found that active bleeding and/or angioectasias were found in 44.4% of inpatients whose VCE was performed within 3 days of their admission for bleeding versus 27.8% when it was performed after 72 hours. Significantly higher rates of therapeutic intervention (18.9% vs 7.4%) and shorter lengths of stay (6.1 days vs 10.3 days) were also seen in the group whose VCE was performed early.[2] A small retrospective study of 68 patients who underwent VCE for overt GI bleeding corroborates that positive findings occur more often when VCE is performed closer to the bleeding event.[9] If clinical suspicion for small bowel bleeding remains high, sometimes VCE needs to be repeated after a negative initial examination.[3,10,11]

Although the diagnostic yield is lower when overt bleeding is absent, VCE is indicated for evaluation of select patients with iron deficiency anemia. Positive findings are more often found when blood transfusions have been required, a patient's hemoglobin level is less than 10 g/dL despite iron replacement, and when anemia has been present for 6 months or longer and the diagnostic yield of VCE in this context ranges from 26% to 66%.[3,12–14]

Clinics care points

- VCE is indicated for the evaluation of suspected overt small bowel bleeding and should be pursued if high quality upper endoscopy and colonoscopy are nondiagnostic.
- In patients with overt bleeding, VCE should be performed as close to the bleeding event as possible.

- VCE has a role in the evaluation of patients with iron deficiency anemia, especially in those who have required blood transfusion, have a hemoglobin level of 10 g/dL or less despite iron replacement, and those who have been anemic for more than 6 months.

CROHN'S DISEASE
Diagnosing Suspected Disease

Crohn's disease is suggested in patients with a combination of clinical symptoms and abnormal objective findings on a range of assessments, including biochemical markers, imaging, and endoscopy.[15,16] There is no gold standard for making the diagnosis of Crohn's disease, but ileocolonoscopy with biopsy and small bowel imaging studies are used most commonly.[16]

VCE is indicated when Crohn's disease is suspected clinically, but ileocolonoscopy and cross-sectional imaging have been nondiagnostic.[3,16] A meta-analysis of 19 trials confirmed the usefulness of using VCE in suspected Crohn's disease, showing it to have a higher diagnostic yield than ileocolonoscopy (47% vs 25%), small bowel radiography (52% vs 16%), and computed tomography enterography (68% vs 21%).[17] Another study showed VCE to be more sensitive and specific for the detection of ileal Crohn's than both computed tomography and MR enterography.[18] When patients have perianal Crohn's disease but no other evident disease on conventional evaluation, VCE can lead to management changes in up to one-quarter of these patients.[19]

VCE is best used when Crohn's disease is suspected because of both symptoms and abnormal biochemical markers or other inflammatory bowel disease-related findings. The yield of VCE is low in patients with abdominal pain and diarrhea alone. A study of 20 patients with chronic abdominal pain and extensive prior negative work-up showed that the use of VCE demonstrated no significant clinical value to any patient case.[20] One multicenter study found that the diagnostic yield of VCE was 66.7% in patients with abdominal pain and positive inflammatory markers (C-reactive protein and erythrocyte sedimentation rate) and 90.1% of patients with abdominal pain, diarrhea, and positive inflammatory markers, but only 21.4% in patients with abdominal pain and negative inflammatory markers and none of the patients with abdominal pain, diarrhea, and negative inflammatory markers.[21] A prospective multicenter trial found the presence of inflammatory markers to have the greatest impact on the diagnostic yield of VCE in this context, with an odds ration of 3.2.[22] A different retrospective study in 70 patients with negative bidirectional endoscopies found that increasing levels of fecal calprotein were good positive predictors of VCE findings of Crohn's disease. All patients with fecal calprotectin levels less than 100 μg/g had normal VCE results whereas 43% of patients with fecal calprotein levels greater than 100 μg/g and 65% of patient with fecal calprotein levels greater than 200 μg/g had positive VCE findings.[23]

Monitoring Established Disease

VCE is indicated in patients with known Crohn's disease who are symptomatic despite having no active inflammatory findings on ileocolonoscopy and imaging studies.[3] A meta-analysis showed that VCE had a higher yield for detecting active inflammation in patients like this than push enteroscopy (66% vs 9%), small bowel radiography (71% vs 36%), and computed tomography enterography (71% vs 39%).[17] Findings on VCE in these patients often results in changes to their management.[24,25]

VCE is also indicated for the detection of active small bowel disease in select asymptomatic patients with known Crohn's disease. Symptom resolution does not always correlate with mucosal healing, but the importance of mucosal healing is becoming an increasingly targeted goal of Crohn's therapies because of its association with higher rates of sustained clinical remission and lower rates of hospitalization and surgery.[3,26–30] Two prospective studies have demonstrated that when VCE was performed in patients who had achieved clinical and biochemical remission with treatment for Crohn's enteritis, 0% had achieved complete mucosal healing by 12 weeks and only 42% had achieved mucosal healing by week 52.[27,28]

VCE can also be used to assess for postoperative recurrence of Crohn's enteritis when ileocolonoscopy and imaging studies have been unrevealing.[3] Although ileocolonoscopy is more sensitive in detecting local recurrence in the neoterminal ileum, VCE detected lesions not seen on ileocolonoscopy in more than two-thirds of patients.[31]

Clinics care points

- VCE is indicated in patients in whom Crohn's disease remains clinically suspected despite negative findings on conventional imaging and ileocolonoscopy and clinical suspicion remains high. The yield in this cohort is higher when objective biochemical markers are also present.
- With emerging data highlighting the importance of achieving mucosal healing with Crohn's therapy, VCE can be used to assess the small bowel mucosa in Crohn's patients who have achieved clinical remission.

CELIAC DISEASE

Celiac disease is an autoimmune condition in which cross-reactivity to gluten results in histologically evident enteropathy. If other appropriate investigations for persistent symptoms are nondiagnostic, VCE is indicated in patients with known celiac disease who remain symptomatic despite the adoption of a gluten-free diet, especially in those with true refractory disease.[3] Given its ability to visualize the mucosal surface of the entire small bowel, VCE has demonstrated that 15% to 30% of patients with refractory celiac disease have pertinent findings including lymphoma, ulcerative jejunitis, and adenocarcinoma.[3,32–34]

The use of VCE to make or refute the diagnosis of celiac disease in equivocal cases remains controversial. In patients with positive serologies but normal duodenal biopsies, VCE likely adds little to the diagnostic process except for cost. In a study of this subset of patients, no patients had mucosal changes consistent with celiac disease on VCE and multiple meta-analyses have demonstrated that VCE after endoscopy with normal duodenal biopsies has a low diagnostic yield.[35,36] There is evidence to support the use of VCE in patients with villous atrophy detected on duodenal biopsy but negative celiac serologies. A recent study of this cohort of patients showed VCE to have a diagnostic yield of 40% on those patients in whom the etiology of their villous atrophy remained unknown before VCE.[37]

Clinics Care Points

- VCE is indicated for the investigation of refractory celiac disease owing to its ability to detect significant complications from this.
- VCE has not been proven useful in patients with positive celiac serologies but normal duodenal biopsies.
- VCE may have a role in patients with seronegative villous atrophy.

POLYPOSIS SYNDROMES

Although most polyposis syndromes manifest primarily with colonic polyps and an escalated risk of colonic malignancy, several syndromes, most notably familial adenomatous polyposis (FAP) and Peutz–Jeghers syndrome, increase the risk for small bowel polyps and small bowel malignancy. VCE is therefore indicated for small bowel surveillance in patients with certain polyposis syndromes.[3] Multiple studies have shown that VCE has greater diagnostic yields when compared with other modalities for the detection of small bowel polyps in these patients. One study demonstrated that 76% of patients with FAP and known duodenal adenomas had additional adenomas in the proximal jejunum detectable by VCE or push enteroscopy and that 24% of these patients had more distal polyps that could only be seen with VCE.[38] VCE has been shown to have a higher yield for polyp detection than barium-based small bowel follow through examinations and MR enterography in patients with FAP or Peutz–Jeghers syndrome.[39,40]

Clinics Care Point

- VCE is indicated for polyp surveillance in patients with polyposis syndromes that can manifest with small bowel lesions, most commonly Peutz–Jeghers syndrome and FAP.

CONTRAINDICATIONS AND CONSIDERATIONS

The only absolute contraindications to VCE are complete or partial esophageal, gastric outlet, and small or large bowel obstruction, but several potential issues must be considered before performing VCE.

Incomplete Examination

To perform a high-quality examination and maximize diagnostic yield, VCE should ideally visualize the entire small bowel. An incomplete examination occurs when the capsule does not reach the cecum before the end of its recording time, something that occurs in 16% to 20% of examinations.[3,41,42] Advancing age, male sex, inpatient status, and suspected or known Crohn's disease are risk factors for an incomplete examination.[41,43] Some data suggest that the rates of complete examination will likely be higher with newer generation capsules, which have increased battery lives of up to 12 hours.[44] Although opioids decrease GI motility, there is no clear evidence that patients on opioids have lower rates of VCE completion.[43,45] Similarly, completion rates have not been found to be clearly lower in patients with impaired gastric emptying, although if delayed gastric passage is expected, endoscopic placement of the video capsule distal to the pylorus will increase the likelihood of a complete examination.[43,46,47] Although data are mixed and studies heterogenous, using metoclopramide in conjunction with a bowel preparation has been shown to increase the likelihood of a complete examination.[48]

CAPSULE RETENTION

Capsule retention, the continued presence of the capsule in the digestive tract for more than 2 weeks, is the most serious complication of VCE. Although the capsule itself is inert, retention can cause obstructive symptoms in up to 22% of patients with retention, and endoscopic or surgical intervention are frequently pursued to retrieve the capsule.[41] The risk of capsule retention is low, occurring in 1.3% to 1.4% of cases performed.[41,42] Similar rates are seen in patients with suspected Crohn's disease (0%

to 1.6%), but much higher retention rates, 5% to 13%, are seen in patients with known Crohn's disease.[41,49,50] In addition to Crohn's, other factors associated with an increased risk of retention are known strictures, a history of abdominopelvic radiation or a suspected tumor.[41,51]

When there is a high preprocedure concern for stricturing and capsule retention, a patency capsule that consists of a biodegradable body surrounding a small radiofrequency identification tag can be considered before performing VCE.[3] Studies have demonstrated that the passage of an intact patency capsule in patients with known or suspected intestinal stricture is predictive of successful passage of the VCE in almost all cases.[52,53] Although designed to quickly and safely biodegrade, patency capsules have been reported to cause abdominal pain and, in rare cases, obstructive symptoms requiring surgery.[52–55] Cross-sectional imaging studies can also be used to predict the patency of bowel for passage of the video capsule with similar sensitivity for predicting clinically significant small bowel strictures as patency capsules.[53,56]

MISSED LESIONS

Like any endoscopic evaluation, VCE is not a perfect study and missed lesions can occur. Because small bowel masses occur infrequently in the general population and negative VCE examinations are not often followed by subsequent device-assisted enteroscopy or repeat VCE, the true risk of missed lesions is uncertain. In 1 retrospective study of 300 VCE examinations performed for GI bleeding, 9 examinations showed masses, one of which had been missed on prior VCE.[57]

PACEMAKERS

VCE manufacturers list the presence of a cardiac pacemaker or other implanted electromedical devices as a contraindication for the use of VCE.[3] Despite this advice, in clinical practice performing VCE in the presence of a pacemaker has been shown to be safe and only rarely is the image acquisition affected.[3] One retrospective study evaluated the safety and transmission quality of VCE in more than 100 patients with implantable electromechanical cardiac devices found no effect of the capsule on the cardiac device. Image acquisition was effected in none of the patients with pacemakers and only 1 patient with an implantable cardioverter-defibrillator and 2 patients with left ventricular assist devices.[58] In another retrospective multicenter study involving 62 VCE examinations, no pacemakers or implantable cardioverter-defibrillators were functionally impaired and only examinations featured interference between the video capsule and telemetry.[59]

Clinics Care Points

- VCE is only contraindicated in patients with known luminal obstruction; however, incomplete studies, capsule retention, and missed lesions can all occur.
- Patients with delayed gut transit time, including those taking narcotics, do not clearly have higher rates of incomplete VCE examinations and are still candidates for VCE examination.
- Multiple techniques, including prokinetics, endoscopic placement of the capsule into the duodenum, and extended battery life video capsules, can be used to increase crates of study completion.
- Patency capsule or cross-sectional imaging can be used in patients with known or suspected strictures of the small bowel to better predict the risk of retention.
- VCE can be performed safely in patients with pacemakers and other implantable cardiac devices without special precautions.

DISCLOSURE

Neither author has any pertinent disclosures.

REFERENCES

1. Lewis BS. Small intestinal bleeding. Gastroenterol Clin North Am 1994;23:67–91.
2. Singh A, Marshall C, Chaudhuri B, et al. Timing of video capsule endoscopy relative to overt obscure GI bleeding: implications from a retrospective study. Gastrointest Endosc 2013;77:761–6.
3. Enns RA, Hookey L, Armstrong D, et al. Clinical practice guidelines for the use of video capsule endoscopy. Gastroenterology 2017;152:497–514.
4. Teshima CW, Kuipers EJ, van Zanten SV, et al. Double balloon enteroscopy and capsule endoscopy for obscure gastrointestinal bleeding: an updated meta-analysis. J Gastroenterol Hepatol 2011;26:796–801.
5. Viazis N, Papaxoinis K, Vlachogiannakos J, et al. Is there a role for second-look capsule endoscopy in patients with obscure GI bleeding after a nondiagnostic first test? Gastrointest Endosc 2009;69:850–6.
6. Laine L, Sahota A, Shah A. Does capsule endoscopy improve outcomes in obscure gastrointestinal bleeding? Randomized trial versus dedicated small bowel radiography. Gastroenterology 2010;138:1673–80.e1 [quiz e11-2].
7. Leung WK, Ho SS, Suen BY, et al. Capsule endoscopy or angiography in patients with acute overt obscure gastrointestinal bleeding: a prospective randomized study with long-term follow-up. Am J Gastroenterol 2012;107:1370–6.
8. Segarajasingam DS, Hanley SC, Barkun AN, et al. Randomized controlled trial comparing outcomes of video capsule endoscopy with push enteroscopy in obscure gastrointestinal bleeding. Can J Gastroenterol Hepatol 2015;29:85–90.
9. Esaki M, Matsumoto T, Yada S, et al. Factors associated with the clinical impact of capsule endoscopy in patients with overt obscure gastrointestinal bleeding. Dig Dis Sci 2010;55:2294–301.
10. Pioche M, Gaudin JL, Filoche B, et al. Prospective, randomized comparison of two small-bowel capsule endoscopy systems in patients with obscure GI bleeding. Gastrointest Endosc 2011;73:1181–8.
11. Min BH, Chang DK, Kim BJ, et al. Does back-to-back capsule endoscopy increase the diagnostic yield over a single examination in patients with obscure gastrointestinal bleeding? Gut Liver 2010;4:54–9.
12. Koulaouzidis A, Rondonotti E, Giannakou A, et al. Diagnostic yield of small-bowel capsule endoscopy in patients with iron-deficiency anemia: a systematic review. Gastrointest Endosc 2012;76:983–92.
13. Koulaouzidis A, Yung DE, Lam JH, et al. The use of small-bowel capsule endoscopy in iron-deficiency anemia alone; be aware of the young anemic patient. Scand J Gastroenterol 2012;47:1094–100.
14. Tong J, Svarta S, Ou G, et al. Diagnostic yield of capsule endoscopy in the setting of iron deficiency anemia without evidence of gastrointestinal bleeding. Can J Gastroenterol 2012;26:687–90.
15. Sands BE. From symptom to diagnosis: clinical distinctions among various forms of intestinal inflammation. Gastroenterology 2004;126:1518–32.
16. Van Assche G, Dignass A, Panes J, et al. The second European evidence-based consensus on the diagnosis and management of Crohn's disease: definitions and diagnosis. J Crohns Colitis 2010;4:7–27.
17. Dionisio PM, Gurudu SR, Leighton JA, et al. Capsule endoscopy has a significantly higher diagnostic yield in patients with suspected and established

small-bowel Crohn's disease: a meta-analysis. Am J Gastroenterol 2010;105: 1240–8 [quiz 1249].

18. Jensen MD, Nathan T, Rafaelsen SR, et al. Diagnostic accuracy of capsule endoscopy for small bowel Crohn's disease is superior to that of MR enterography or CT enterography. Clin Gastroenterol Hepatol 2011;9:124–9.

19. Adler SN, Yoav M, Eitan S, et al. Does capsule endoscopy have an added value in patients with perianal disease and a negative work up for Crohn's disease? World J Gastrointest Endosc 2012;4:185–8.

20. Bardan E, Nadler M, Chowers Y, et al. Capsule endoscopy for the evaluation of patients with chronic abdominal pain. Endoscopy 2003;35:688–9.

21. Katsinelos P, Fasoulas K, Beltsis A, et al. Diagnostic yield and clinical impact of wireless capsule endoscopy in patients with chronic abdominal pain with or without diarrhea: a Greek multicenter study. Eur J Intern Med 2011;22:e63–6.

22. May A, Manner H, Schneider M, et al. Prospective multicenter trial of capsule endoscopy in patients with chronic abdominal pain, diarrhea and other signs and symptoms (CEDAP-Plus Study). Endoscopy 2007;39:606–12.

23. Koulaouzidis A, Douglas S, Rogers MA, et al. Fecal calprotectin: a selection tool for small bowel capsule endoscopy in suspected IBD with prior negative bidirectional endoscopy. Scand J Gastroenterol 2011;46:561–6.

24. Voderholzer WA, Beinhoelzl J, Rogalla P, et al. Small bowel involvement in Crohn's disease: a prospective comparison of wireless capsule endoscopy and computed tomography enteroclysis. Gut 2005;54:369–73.

25. Lorenzo-Zuniga V, de Vega VM, Domenech E, et al. Impact of capsule endoscopy findings in the management of Crohn's disease. Dig Dis Sci 2010;55:411–4.

26. Efthymiou A, Viazis N, Mantzaris G, et al. Does clinical response correlate with mucosal healing in patients with Crohn's disease of the small bowel? A prospective, case-series study using wireless capsule endoscopy. Inflamm Bowel Dis 2008;14:1542–7.

27. Hall BJ, Holleran GE, Smith SM, et al. A prospective 12-week mucosal healing assessment of small bowel Crohn's disease as detected by capsule endoscopy. Eur J Gastroenterol Hepatol 2014;26:1253–9.

28. Hall B, Holleran G, Chin JL, et al. A prospective 52 week mucosal healing assessment of small bowel Crohn's disease as detected by capsule endoscopy. J Crohns Colitis 2014;8:1601–9.

29. Lichtenstein GR, Loftus EV, Isaacs KL, et al. ACG clinical guideline: management of Crohn's disease in adults. Am J Gastroenterol 2018;113:481–517.

30. Picco MF, Farraye FA. Targeting mucosal healing in Crohn's disease. Gastroenterol Hepatol (N Y) 2019;15:529–38.

31. Bourreille A, Jarry M, D'Halluin PN, et al. Wireless capsule endoscopy versus ileocolonoscopy for the diagnosis of postoperative recurrence of Crohn's disease: a prospective study. Gut 2006;55:978–83.

32. Atlas DS, Rubio-Tapia A, Van Dyke CT, et al. Capsule endoscopy in nonresponsive celiac disease. Gastrointest Endosc 2011;74:1315–22.

33. Kurien M, Evans KE, Aziz I, et al. Capsule endoscopy in adult celiac disease: a potential role in equivocal cases of celiac disease? Gastrointest Endosc 2013;77: 227–32.

34. Barret M, Malamut G, Rahmi G, et al. Diagnostic yield of capsule endoscopy in refractory celiac disease. Am J Gastroenterol 2012;107:1546–53.

35. El-Matary W, Huynh H, Vandermeer B. Diagnostic characteristics of given video capsule endoscopy in diagnosis of celiac disease: a meta-analysis. J Laparoendosc Adv Surg Tech A 2009;19:815–20.

36. Rokkas T, Niv Y. The role of video capsule endoscopy in the diagnosis of celiac disease: a meta-analysis. Eur J Gastroenterol Hepatol 2012;24:303–8.
37. Chetcuti Zammit S, Schiepatti A, Aziz I, et al. Use of small-bowel capsule endoscopy in cases of equivocal celiac disease. Gastrointest Endosc 2020;91: 1312–21.e2.
38. Schulmann K, Hollerbach S, Kraus K, et al. Feasibility and diagnostic utility of video capsule endoscopy for the detection of small bowel polyps in patients with hereditary polyposis syndromes. Am J Gastroenterol 2005;100:27–37.
39. Mata A, Llach J, Castells A, et al. A prospective trial comparing wireless capsule endoscopy and barium contrast series for small-bowel surveillance in hereditary GI polyposis syndromes. Gastrointest Endosc 2005;61:721–5.
40. Tescher P, Macrae FA, Speer T, et al. Surveillance of FAP: a prospective blinded comparison of capsule endoscopy and other GI imaging to detect small bowel polyps. Hered Cancer Clin Pract 2010;8:3.
41. Höög CM, Bark L, Arkani J, et al. Capsule retentions and incomplete capsule endoscopy examinations: an analysis of 2300 examinations. Gastroenterol Res Pract 2012;2012:518718.
42. Liao Z, Gao R, Xu C, et al. Indications and detection, completion, and retention rates of small-bowel capsule endoscopy: a systematic review. Gastrointest Endosc 2010;71:280–6.
43. Yazici C, Losurdo J, Brown MD, et al. Inpatient capsule endoscopy leads to frequent incomplete small bowel examinations. World J Gastroenterol 2012;18: 5051–7.
44. Ou G, Shahidi N, Galorport C, et al. Effect of longer battery life on small bowel capsule endoscopy. World J Gastroenterol 2015;21:2677–82.
45. Lee MM, Jacques A, Lam E, et al. Factors associated with incomplete small bowel capsule endoscopy studies. World J Gastroenterol 2010;16:5329–33.
46. Shiotani A, Honda K, Kawakami M, et al. Use of an external real-time image viewer coupled with prespecified actions enhanced the complete examinations for capsule endoscopy. J Gastroenterol Hepatol 2011;26:1270–4.
47. Hoog CM, Lindberg G, Sjoqvist U. Findings in patients with chronic intestinal dysmotility investigated by capsule endoscopy. BMC Gastroenterol 2007;7:29.
48. Koulaouzidis A, Giannakou A, Yung DE, et al. Do prokinetics influence the completion rate in small-bowel capsule endoscopy? A systematic review and meta-analysis. Curr Med Res Opin 2013;29:1171–85.
49. Cheifetz AS, Kornbluth AA, Legnani P, et al. The risk of retention of the capsule endoscope in patients with known or suspected Crohn's disease. Am J Gastroenterol 2006;101:2218–22.
50. Atay O, Mahajan L, Kay M, et al. Risk of capsule endoscope retention in pediatric patients: a large single-center experience and review of the literature. J Pediatr Gastroenterol Nutr 2009;49:196–201.
51. Singeap AM, Trifan A, Cojocariu C, et al. Outcomes after symptomatic capsule retention in suspected small bowel obstruction. Eur J Gastroenterol Hepatol 2011;23:886–90.
52. Banerjee R, Bhargav P, Reddy P, et al. Safety and efficacy of the M2A patency capsule for diagnosis of critical intestinal patency: results of a prospective clinical trial. J Gastroenterol Hepatol 2007;22:2060–3.
53. Boivin ML, Lochs H, Voderholzer WA. Does passage of a patency capsule indicate small-bowel patency? A prospective clinical trial? Endoscopy 2005;37: 808–15.

54. Postgate AJ, Burling D, Gupta A, et al. Safety, reliability and limitations of the given patency capsule in patients at risk of capsule retention: a 3-year technical review. Dig Dis Sci 2008;53:2732–8.

55. Herrerias JM, Leighton JA, Costamagna G, et al. Agile patency system eliminates risk of capsule retention in patients with known intestinal strictures who undergo capsule endoscopy. Gastrointest Endosc 2008;67:902–9.

56. Yadav A, Heigh RI, Hara AK, et al. Performance of the patency capsule compared with nonenteroclysis radiologic examinations in patients with known or suspected intestinal strictures. Gastrointest Endosc 2011;74:834–9.

57. Baichi MM, Arifuddin RM, Mantry PS. Small-bowel masses found and missed on capsule endoscopy for obscure bleeding. Scand J Gastroenterol 2007;42:1127–32.

58. Harris LA, Hansel SL, Rajan E, et al. Capsule endoscopy in patients with implantable electromedical devices is safe. Gastroenterol Res Pract 2013;2013:959234.

59. Bandorski D, Lotterer E, Hartmann D, et al. Capsule endoscopy in patients with cardiac pacemakers and implantable cardioverter-defibrillators - a retrospective multicenter investigation. J Gastrointest Liver Dis 2011;20:33–7.

Role of Video Capsule in Small Bowel Bleeding

Richard M. Wu, MD, MPH[a], Laurel R. Fisher, MD[b],*

KEYWORDS

- Gastrointestinal bleeding • Suspected small bowel bleeding • Angioectasias
- GI angiodysplasia Video capsule endoscopy • Small bowel hemorrhagic lesions
- Small bowel tumors • Small bowel ulcers

KEY POINTS

- Small bowel bleeding accounts for 5% to 10% of all gastrointestinal bleeding and video capsule endoscopy is the first-line study recommended study for this condition.
- Video capsule endoscopy diagnostic yields differ depending on indication. The highest yield occurs in overt suspected small bowel bleeding, especially if video capsule endoscopy is performed within 3 days of the incident bleeding episode.
- Multiple etiologies of small bowel bleeding can be detected on video capsule endoscopy.
- The role of video capsule endoscopy in small bowel bleeding is broad and includes assessment of iron deficiency anemia and acute and chronic blood loss.
- Future roles will be enhanced by the incorporation of magnet technology and artificial intelligence.

INTRODUCTION AND VIDEO CAPSULE ENDOSCOPY USE

Gastrointestinal (GI) bleeding has accounted for more than 500,000 admissions yearly in the United States.[1] Colonoscopy and esophagogastroduodenoscopy (EGD) identify the cause of blood loss in the majority of patients with GI bleeding, but in 5% to 10% of cases, the source is found in the small bowel.

In the last 20 years, the small bowel has become accessible by newer technologies, most dramatically by small bowel video capsule endoscopy (VCE) and subsequently by device-assisted enteroscopy or dedicated radiologic imaging. VCE is now considered the first-line diagnostic study for small bowel bleeding.

Since the initial approval by the US Food and Drug Administration of the GIVEN imaging VCE device in 2001, 5 other small bowel devices have been developed world

---

[a] Division of Gastroenterology and Hepatology, Corporal Michael J. Crescenz Veterans Affairs Medical Center, University of Pennsylvania Health System, 4th Floor GI Department, 3900 Woodland Avenue, Philadelphia, PA 19104, USA; [b] Small Bowel Imaging Program, Division of Gastroenterology and Hepatology, University of Pennsylvania Health System, 3400 Civic Center Drive, PCAM 7S, Philadelphia, PA 19104, USA
* Corresponding author.
E-mail address: Laurel.fisher@pennmedicine.penn.edu

Gastrointest Endoscopy Clin N Am 31 (2021) 277–306
https://doi.org/10.1016/j.giec.2020.12.003
1052-5157/21/© 2020 Elsevier Inc. All rights reserved.

giendo.theclinics.com

wide: in the United States—EndoCam (Olympus, Tokyo, Japan; 2008), MiroCam (IntroMedic, Goru-gu, South Korea, 2012), and CapsoCam (CapsoVision, Saratoga, CA, 2016); and internationally—Omom (Jinshan Science and Technology, Chongqing, China 2004) and Sayaka (RF Systems, Nagano, Japan). The overall global capsule endoscopy market is expected to grow to 1.30 billion USD by 2026.[2] What was once considered a unique disruptive technology is now standard of care for small bowel evaluation. Although VCE is approved by the US Food and Drug Administration for assessment of Crohn's disease and iron deficiency anemia (IDA), and is used in numerous settings, its primary approved indication remains the evaluation of small bowel bleeding.

GUIDELINES FOR USE

Guidelines of the American College of Gastroenterology,[3] the American Society of Gastrointestinal Endoscopy,[4] and the American Gastroenterological Association[5] affirm VCE as the first-line study for small bowel bleeding in hemodynamically stable patients. VCE delivers a high diagnostic yield compared with other technologies, although widely ranging from 38% to 87%.[6,7] What was previously termed "obscure GI bleeding" has been reclassified as "small bowel bleeding" and the term "obscure GI bleeding" is now reserved for bleeding whose source is not identified after bidirectional endoscopy and small bowel evaluation.

Algorithms

The GI societies have designed algorithms to guide clinicians in the appropriate evaluation of small bowel bleeding. Early algorithms strategized by occult versus overt GI bleeding (**Fig. 1**)[3,8] but more recent decision trees begin with hemodynamic status (**Fig. 2**).[9] Another management strategy suggests that further clinical decisions be based on major, minor, or absent findings on initial VCE.[10] All algorithms, however, recommend endoscopic evaluation with EGD and colonoscopy before consideration of a small bowel source, and all introduce caution before VCE use in patients with potential for small bowel obstruction.

After first-line use of VCE, algorithmic direction for small bowel bleeding is less well-defined, and multiple options are available.

- For patients with positive identification of a small bowel bleeding source by VCE, direct therapy is recommended. In general, for patients in this category who re-bleed, it is recommended that therapy be directed toward the known lesion.
- For stable patients with a negative VCE, conservative therapy can be followed. Although false negatives occur,[11] a conservative approach is supported by many practitioners. A meta-analysis concluded that a negative VCE confers low risk of rebleeding,[12] suggesting that patients can frequently be managed with oral iron and observation.

Recurrence of Small Bowel Bleeding

The rebleeding rate after an initial negative VCE range from 5% to 25%,[12,13] and for patients with prior positive findings on VCE, 30% to 40% may rebleed.

Consensus statements recommend no specific pathway for recurrent bleeders. Acceptable options include repeat bidirectional endoscopy, and/or VCE, or other imaging modalities such as computed tomography angiography, depending on the clinical setting and physician judgment. The rationale for repeat bidirectional endoscopy includes data showing that approximately one-quarter of sites of rebleeding are in

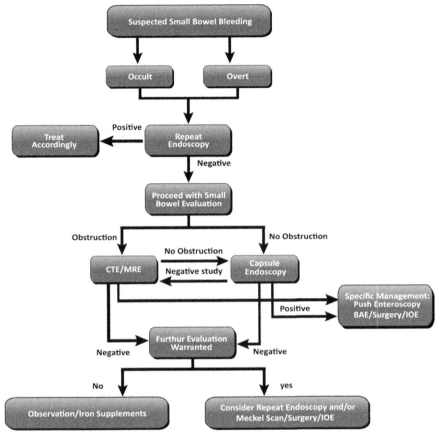

Fig. 1. Suspected small bowel bleeding algorithm stratified by overt versus occult. BAE, Balloon Assisted Enteroscopy; IOE, Intraoperative enteroscopy. (*From*: Gerson LB, Fidler JL, Cave DR, Leighton JA. ACG Clinical Guideline: Diagnosis and Management of Small Bowel Bleeding. *Am J Gastroenterol.* 2015;110(9):1265-1287; with permission.)

reach of the endoscope.[14] Device-assisted enteroscopy is an option, although the lack of a target lesion diminishes the yield severely.

Repeat VCE for patients who rebleed should be considered for a decrease in hemoglobin of more than 4 g, a change from occult to overt bleeding, or the development of severe IDA with a hemoglobin of less than 10 g/dL.[15] Predictors of a positive initial or repeat small bowel study for recurrent bleeding are described in **Table 1**.

One long-term follow-up study of "obscure" GI bleeding noted the rebleeding rate after VCE to be higher for patients with a previous positive VCE study without treatment, (47.6%) and lower after specific therapy (25.7%) or a negative study (20.8%).[16]

According to 1 multivariate analysis, ongoing overt GI bleeding and severe anemia at initial VCE examination were independent factors associated with rebleeding in patients with overt "obscure" GI bleeding.[17]

Timing of Video Capsule Endoscopy in Gastrointestinal Bleeding

Algorithms do not address the timing of VCE. Expert consensus favors initiation of a VCE evaluation as soon as possible to increase the diagnostic yield. Early studies

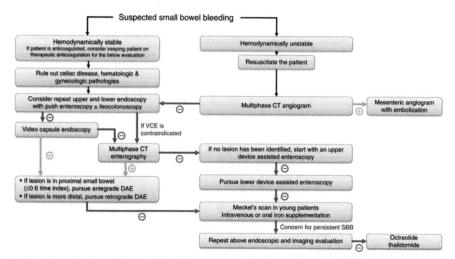

Fig. 2. Suspected small bowel bleeding stratified by hemodynamic stability. CT, computed tomography; DAE, Device Assisted Enteroscopy. (*From*: Kuo JR, Pasha SF, Leighton JA. The Clinician's Guide to Suspected Small Bowel Bleeding. *Am J Gastroenterol.* 2019;114(4):591-598; with permission.)

recommended a 2-week window, but more current data demonstrate that VCE closer to the event leads to a higher diagnostic yield (44%–91%).[5,18–20] One study comparing inpatient VCE before and after 3 days of hospitalization and outpatient VCE supports its use within 72 hours for the optimization of diagnostic and therapeutic yield, and for a decrease in length of hospital stay.[18] Timely inpatient VCE procedures may increase yield by expediting timing,[21] but outpatient examinations are likely to be more complete.[22]

DISCUSSION
Clinical and Endoscopic View of Small Bowel Hemorrhagic Lesions

Findings associated with small bowel bleeding
What are the video capsule endoscopy findings associated with gastrointestinal bleeding?. Small bowel hemorrhagic lesions can be categorized as primary vascular

Table 1	
Positive predictors of a small bowel bleeding study	
Initial Bleeding	**Recurrent Bleeding**
Active overt > inactive overt	Decline in hemoglobin >4 g
Overt > occult bleeding	Prior lesion on enteroscopy
Short timeframe from initial bleed	Change from occult to overt bleeding
Severe anemia	IDA with decline in hemoglobin to <10 g
Increasing transfusion requirements	
Multiple recurrent bleeding episodes	

Adapted from Viazis N, Papaxoinis K, Vlachogiannakos J, et al. Is there a role for second-look capsule endoscopy in patients with obscure GI bleeding after a nondiagnostic first test? *Gastrointest Endosc.* 2009;69(4):850-856; Techima, Christopher *Obscure Gastrointestinal Bleeding,* Endoscopy in Small Bowel Disorders, Kozarek, Leighton, Ed, Springer Publishing, NY, 2015, p. 127-139; with permission.

(small or large vessel), or nonvascular lesions, including infiltrative, mechanical, ulcerative, inflammatory, or neoplastic lesions. The prevalence of these lesions in one study was 50% for vascular lesions, 27% for inflammation and ulcers, 9% for neoplasm, 7% for bleeding, and 8% for other causes.[23]

Patients with older than 60 years of age have a higher prevalence of angioectasias, ulcerative lesions, and nonsteroidal anti-inflammatory drug–related enteropathy and those less than 50 years of age have a higher incidence of Crohn's disease and Meckel's diverticulum.[24] Other clinical risk factors associated with higher VCE diagnostic yield include connective tissue disease, cirrhosis, renal disease, cardiac valvular disease, left ventricular assist device (LVAD), anticoagulation, greater transfusion requirements, and overt bleeding.[25,26]

Small bowel lesions have different hemorrhagic risks. With the use of a classification system such as the Saurin system, which identifies lesion characteristics, VCE can be used to predict the impending risk of bleeding (**Table 2**).[27] P2 lesions, including classical angioectasia, large ulcers, tumor, and varices, have a high bleeding probability. P1 lesions, including red spots and small aphthous ulcers, have a less well-defined, low to intermediate bleeding probability. P0 lesions, including submucosal veins, nonbleeding diverticula, and small nodules, are not associated with bleeding.

Vascular lesions
Small vessel vascular lesions
    What is the most common cause of small bowel bleeding seen on video capsule endoscopy? Small vessel vascular lesions are the most common VCE finding.[28] The term "gastrointestinal angiodysplasia" erroneously suggests dysplastic histology, therefore making "angioectasia" the preferred term. Other nomenclature includes arteriovenous malformation, vascular ectasia, and telangiectasia. A subclassification was proposed by Yano and colleagues[29] that separates the lesions into 6 groups with the intent of providing recommendations for differential therapeutic endoscopic methods (**Fig. 3**).

Angioectasias (**Fig. 4**) are dilated endothelial vessels between veins and capillaries, lacking a smooth muscle cell layer and susceptible to rupture. The proposed pathophysiology includes mucosal ischemia and hypoxia secondary to chronic venous obstruction and the presence of endothelial growth factors.[30] Angioectasias account for 50% to 60% of obscure GI bleeding etiologies in VCE studies and have a 50% spontaneous bleeding cessation rate.[31] This episodic nature of the bleeding often poses a VCE diagnostic challenge, especially if the VCE procedure is delayed, which may lead to missed culprit lesions. More than 50% of patients will have more than 1 angioectasia lesion and groupings tend to occur anatomically. Bleeding can be mild

Table 2
Saurin classification of small bowel lesions' bleeding potential

Saurin Class	Bleeding Risk	Examples
P0	None	Visible mucosal veins, diverticula without bleeding stigmata, nodules without mucosal breaks
P1	Low	Mucosal red spots, small or isolated erosions
P2	High	Typical angiomata, large ulcers, tumors or varices

Adapted from Saurin JC, Delvaux M, Gaudin JL, et al. Diagnostic value of endoscopic capsule in patients with obscure digestive bleeding: blinded comparison with video push-enteroscopy. *Endoscopy.* 2003;35(7):576-584; with permission.

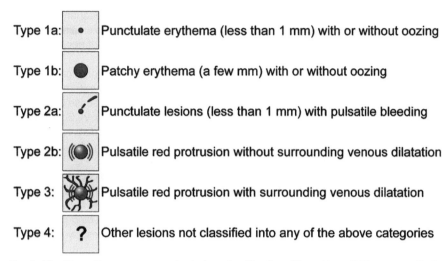

Type 1a: Punctulate erythema (less than 1 mm) with or without oozing

Type 1b: Patchy erythema (a few mm) with or without oozing

Type 2a: Punctulate lesions (less than 1 mm) with pulsatile bleeding

Type 2b: Pulsatile red protrusion without surrounding venous dilatation

Type 3: Pulsatile red protrusion with surrounding venous dilatation

Type 4: ? Other lesions not classified into any of the above categories

Fig. 3. The Yano–Yamamoto vascular lesion classification. (*From* Yano T, Yamamoto H, Sunada K, et al. Endoscopic classification of vascular lesions of the small intestine (with videos). *Gastrointest Endosc.* 2008;67(1):169-172 with permission.)

with associated oozing with small clots (Video 1) or severe active hemorrhage with blood obscuring the underlying vascular lesion (Video 2).

The endoscopic appearance of classic angioectasias is a flat red sharply demarcated fern-like lesion with a central vessel. Enhanced and embedded imaging techniques such as flexible spectral imaging color enhancement can increase the detection rates of angioectasia and can help to discriminate between angioectasias or red spots and inflammatory erosions.[32,33] VCE findings guide the direction of endoscopic treatment of these lesions.[34] Surgery, interventional radiology, and medical therapy with somatostatin analogues and thalidomide may be used for severe or refractory or recurrent bleeding.[35,36]

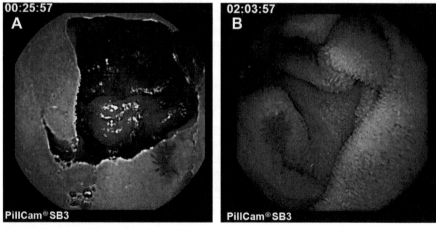

Fig. 4. Classic small bowel angioectasias.

What is Heyde syndrome and how is it managed? Heyde syndrome is a clinical association seen in patients with severe aortic stenosis and VCE-detected GI bleeding.[37] Bleeding from right colon and small bowel angioectasia is likely from a secondary von Willebrand syndrome attributed to the mechanical shear forces of a stenotic aortic valve and an age-related degeneration in the intestinal microcirculation.[38] Approximately 80% of patients will experience cessation of chronic GI bleeding after aortic valve repair.[39]

What is the bleeding risk of a red spot? A common small vessel vascular lesion is the P1 red spot (**Fig. 5**).[26] Red spots are the size of a single villus and are linked to hormonal influences as well as nonsteroidal anti-inflammatory drug use.[40] They have an uncertain bleeding potential; however, given the often intermittent cadence of small bowel bleeding, real-time VCE imaging can occasionally reveal the potential bleeding tendency of red spots, and full dismissal of these lesions needs to be considered carefully, especially if there is trace heme in the region (Video 3).

What are the findings in hereditary hemorrhagic telangiectasia? Hereditary hemorrhagic telangiectasia, or Osler–Weber–Rendu syndrome, is a genetic disorder with multiorgan system arteriovenous malformation and blood vessel fragility, which frequently presents with epistaxis and GI bleeding, most commonly from a gastroduodenal or colonic source. However, IDA owing to small bowel bleeding is common, especially in patients older than 40 years of age. Although active bleeding can be seen in more than 30% of VCE studies in patients with hereditary hemorrhagic telangiectasia, rarely does overt clinical massive bleeding occur.[41] VCE has a diagnostic yield of 70% to 80% and helps to gauge the burden of vascular lesions and guide management decisions and therapeutic planning.[42]

What are the small bowel manifestations of Klippel–Trenaunay–Weber syndrome? Klippel–Trenaunay–Weber syndrome is a congenital vascular syndrome with cutaneous hemangioma, soft tissue hypertrophy, and capillary–venous–lymphatic vascular malformations. Most bleeding is colonic in etiology, and the severity ranges from subtle to overt large-volume bleeding; however, small bowel

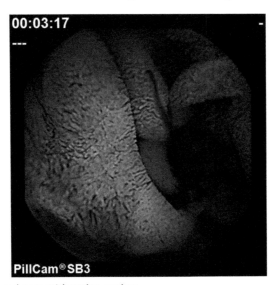

Fig. 5. Saurin P1 red spot with active oozing.

vascular malformations and varices can be seen on VCE in Klippel–Trenaunay–Weber syndrome, resulting in massive GI bleeding.[43]

Large vessel vascular lesions

What are the video capsule endoscopy findings of a Dieulafoy's lesion? A Dieulafoy lesion is a protruding large-caliber submucosal artery without overlying mucosal ulceration. The proximal jejunum is the most common small bowel location. These lesions can bleed profusely, but stop spontaneously **(Fig. 6)**.[44] Given the relatively normal overlying mucosa, they are difficult to identify with VCE during periods of nonbleeding.[45] The first-line treatment is endoscopic hemostasis, but the rebleeding rate is approximately 20%.[46]

What are the video capsule endoscopy findings of small bowel varices? Small bowel varices (SBV) are rare ectopic tortuous venous vessel enlargement found almost exclusively in patients with portal hypertension. SBV are predominantly localized in the duodenum but can occur in the mid to distal small bowel. The endoscopic appearance on VCE may be described as a serpiginous, nodular fold with a bluish coloration, although the mucosal color of SBV may differ minimally from that of the surrounding mucosa **(Fig. 7)**. Adjacent erythema, petechial lesions, or fresh blood and clots may accompany the lesions and help to support the lesions as likely GI bleeding sources. SBV have also been associated with surgical anastomoses and mesenteric vein thrombosis **(Fig. 8)**.[47]

What are the findings in blue rubber bleb nevus syndrome? Blue rubber bleb nevus syndrome is a rare condition characterized by skin, GI viscera, and small bowel venous malformations with chronic recurrent IDA or overt GI bleeding. Uncommon presentations include massive GI bleeding, intussusception, and volvulus. VCE appearance consists of multiple pink, blue, or purple submucosal polypoid lesions ranging 1 to 2 cm in size **(Fig. 9)**.[48,49]

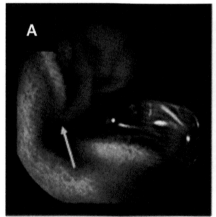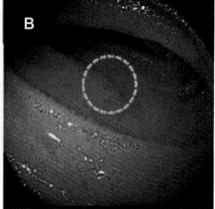

Fig. 6. Actively bleeding Dieulafoy's lesion seen on VCE (*arrow, A*); lesion (mildly protuberant aberrant vessel with cessation of bleeding, dotted circle) seen on double balloon enteroscopy (*B*). (*From* Maeda, Y., Moribata, K., Deguchi, H. *et al.* Video capsule endoscopy as the initial examination for overt obscure gastrointestinal bleeding can efficiently identify patients who require double-balloon enteroscopy. *BMC Gastroenterol* 15, 132 (2015); with permission.)

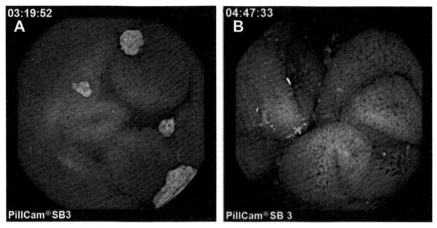

Fig. 7. SBV visualized with VCE.

Nonvascular hemorrhagic lesions
Mechanical lesions
    How common is small bowel diverticulosis and how often do diverticula bleed? Small bowel diverticula occur in 1% to 2% of the population and are localized mostly in the duodenum, followed by the jejunum and ileum. Bleeding from small bowel diverticula is uncommon. Rare cases of episodic diverticular bleeding can be seen (**Fig. 10**), which occurs more frequently in diverticula located in the jejunum and ileum.[50] On VCE, shallow yellowish erosions or ulcerations of the diverticulum apex or peridiverticular area can be seen. VCE findings include a duo lumen with a septum between the lumen and the diverticulum, perpendicular folds, or regional transit delay. In the setting of overt GI bleeding seen on VCE, the accumulation of fresh blood can often obscure the true site of bleeding.[51]

    What are the video capsule endoscopy findings of Meckel's diverticulum? Meckel's diverticulum occurs in 2% to 4% of the population and is typically located at the anti-mesenteric side of the ileum, within 60 cm of the terminal ileum. Bleeding, typically painless, is more common in younger patients. Ulcerated bleeding from the

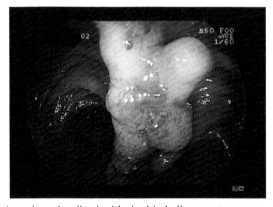

Fig. 8. Anastomotic varices visualized with double balloon enteroscopy.

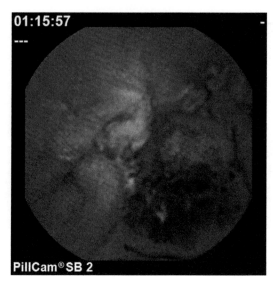

Fig. 9. Blue rubber bleb nevus syndrome.

antidiverticular mucosa can occur.[52] Uncommonly, a large diverticulum can cause a localized appearance of a subepithelial bulge (**Fig. 11**).[53] Three percent of Meckel's diverticulum may have associated tumor transformation.

Infiltrative lesions

Can an intestinal lymphangiectasia be a culprit small bowel bleeding lesion? Nodular lymphangiectasia appearance ranges from multiple small, white, "snow-covered" mucosa findings to larger yellowish mucosal cauliflower-like or submucosal well circumscribed lesions on VCE. These are considered P0 lesions; however, VCE findings of hemorrhagic stippling, discrete red spots (**Fig. 12**), and slow mucosal oozing, can be uncommon sources of small or large volumes of bleeding.[54–56] Microcystic lymphangiectasia (Video 4) are more prone to bleed than macrocystic lymphangiectasia.[57]

How does amyloid contribute to small bowel bleeding? Small bowel amyloidosis occurs when abnormal amyloid protein deposits on the intestinal mucosa form mucosal lesions that can ulcerate and bleed. Small bowel deposits can form thickened folds, erosions, ulcerations, amyloidomas, and submucosal hematoma that lead to IDA or overt small bowel bleeding in up to 40% to 50% of patients (**Fig. 13**).[58]

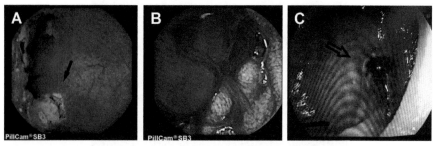

Fig. 10. Mild Mucosal Ulceration (closed arrow) within a jejunal diverticulum on VCE (*A*) and subsequent hemorrhage (*B*), and double balloon enteroscopy showing a visible vessel with active clot (open arrow) at the diverticular apex (*C*).

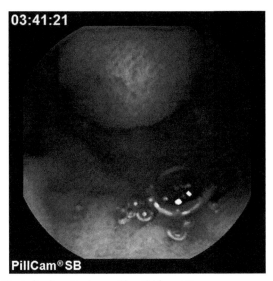

Fig. 11. Inverted Meckel's diverticulum with mild hematin.

Ulcerative and inflammatory lesions

What are the common causes of small bowel ulcerations? A wide range of small intestinal ulcerations can cause IDA and blood loss. Although VCE is an excellent modality for the identification of small bowel ulcerations, the etiology of these lesions can only be determined in the context of clinical history, histology, and/or radiology (Video 5). The most common causes of small bowel ulceration include (**Table 3**) Crohn's disease, celiac disease, nonsteroidal anti-inflammatory drugs, ischemic enteritis, Bechet's disease, tuberculosis, and small bowel tumors.

Crohn's disease: how does it cause bleeding and anemia? Small intestinal Crohn's disease occurs in 80% of patients with Crohn's disease and is characterized by transmural inflammation and ulcerations in a skipped pattern of distribution. Anemia in

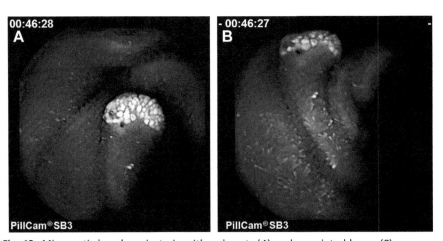

Fig. 12. Microcystic lymphangiectasia with red spots (*A*) and associated heme (*B*).

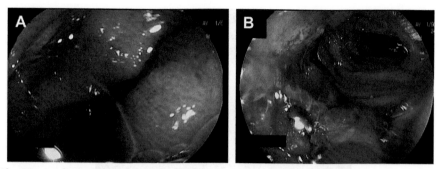

Fig. 13. Amyloid subepithelial mass (A) with overt hemorrhage and clots (B).

Crohn's disease is multifactorial, and luminal bleeding etiologies include subacute chronic blood loss at the ulceration sites and diffuse inflammation.[59]

Lesions found on VCE causing mild anemia include mucosal denudement and aphthous ulcerations. More severe endoscopic findings associated with bleeding include large ulcers (Video 6),[60,61] strictures (**Fig. 14**), pseudopolyps, and rare complications of small bowel adenocarcinoma development.[62] Massive overt hemorrhage can occur with the erosion of a deep ulcer into an adjacent vessel.[63,64]

What celiac disease complications lead to small bowel bleeding? Ulcerative jejunitis, a rare complication of celiac disease, can cause abdominal pain and small bowel bleeding (**Fig. 15**).[65] Refractory celiac disease type II predisposes to a risk of enteropathy-associated T-cell lymphoma and associated overt GI bleeding (Video 7).[66]

Do nonsteroidal anti-inflammatory drug–induced ulcerative lesions cause bleeding? Although nonsteroidal anti-inflammatory drug damage is most often associated with gastric or duodenal lesions, the small bowel is vulnerable to injury resulting in impaired perfusion, ulceration, and bleeding. Early capsule studies in healthy volunteers found IDA or occult bleeding in 1% to 2% of patients, and asymptomatic nonsteroidal anti-inflammatory drug injury in 50% to 70% of patients after as little as 2 weeks of use.[67] VCE findings include erythematous folds (35%), mucosal breaks (40%), petechiae or red spots (33%), denuded mucosa (20%), or active bleeding (5%–8%).[68] The classic multiple, concentric, thin, septa-like diaphragmatic strictures are end-stage

Table 3	
Etiologies of small bowel ulceration	
Etiology	**Examples**
Infectious	CMV, tuberculosis, Yersinia
Infiltrative	Neoplasm, amyloid
Inflammatory	Crohn's disease, vasculitis, radiation, eosinophilic gastroenteritis, Bechet's
Ischemic	Ischemic enteritis, Anastomotic ulcer
Immune related	Celiac disease related ulcerative jejunitis
Medication	NSAIDs, potassium chloride, proton pump inhibitors, chemotherapeutic agents
Congenital	Meckel's
Idiopathic	Chronic enteropathy associated with the *SLCO2A1* gene, cryptogenetic multifocal ulcerous stenosing enteritis

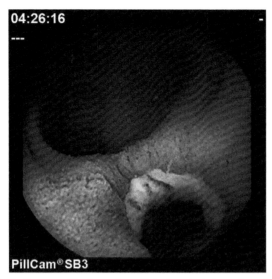

Fig. 14. Ileal Crohn's disease with circumferential ulcerated stenosis and luminal dilation.

pathognomonic findings associated with ulcerations and narrowing, but not bleeding (Video 8).[69]

What other uncommon small bowel enteropathies cause GI bleeding? Ischemic enteritis is attributed to low perfusion of the small bowel ameliorated by rich mesenteric collateral circulation. Subtle blood loss is uncommon and overt GI bleeding is rare. Bechet's disease is a systemic multiorgan disease characterized by oral–genital ulcerations with a 3% to 16% prevalence in the small bowel. VCE findings of erythematous mucosa, erosions, and ulcers are common but nonspecific.[70] The terminal ileal ulcers are can be oval shaped, deep, and punched out appearing.[71] IDA is the most common manifestation but massive GI bleeding has been reported. Tuberculosis-related ulcerations occur mostly in the region of the ileocecal valve and terminal ileum. Tuberculosis ulcers are generally transverse or oblique with

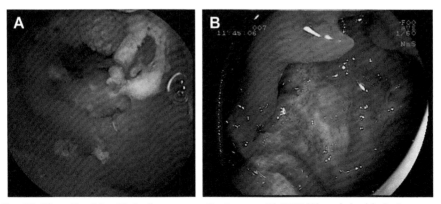

Fig. 15. Ulcerative jejunitis in the same patient seen with VCE (*A*) and double balloon enteroscopy (*B*).

nodularity and a necrotic base that can be hypertrophic and mass like.[72] These ulcerations can cause bowel obstruction, subtle GI blood loss and rare cases of massive ileal bleeding.[73,74]

Neoplastic lesions

What types of small bowel neoplastic lesions contribute to bleeding? Small bowel tumors have seen a gradual rise in incidence from 1 to 2 per 100,000 in the past 2 decades,[75] which correlates with an increase in advanced small bowel imaging such as VCE. Their prevalence in a large multicenter European study was 2.4%.[76] Primary malignant small bowel tumor subtypes are adenocarcinomas (30%–45%), carcinoids (20%–44%), lymphomas (15%–20%) sarcomas (11%–13%), and metastasis (3%–8%). Small bowel tumors account for 5% to 10% of small bowel bleeding etiology.[77]

Small bowel tumors are often slow growing and exhibit variable nonspecific symptoms of bloating, constipation, weight loss, IDA, occult bleeding, and more dramatically, bowel obstruction or overt massive bleeding. Cross-sectional imaging can complement VCE when there is a high suspicion of small bowel neoplasm. There is a 10% to 20% false-negative rate for subtle nonbleeding nonulcerated tumors lesions on VCE studies, especially for proximal small bowel lesions.[78,79]

The VCE features of small bowel submucosal lesions include mucosal disruptions, bleeding, an irregular surface, polypoid appearance, white villi, bridging folds, and invagination. Other diagnostic tools exist, including the SPICE lesion index[80] and mucosal protrusion angulation measurement of the lesion.[81] Machine learning with a convoluted neural network has shown good promise to augment the reader's ability to detect these lesions as well.[82]

Small bowel tumors can be classified as benign lesions versus malignant lesions.

Benign tumors

Are benign tumor sources of small bowel bleeding? Thirty percent to 40% of the small bowel tumors are benign. These tumors include inflammatory or hyperplastic lesions or polyps, ectopic tissues, hamartomas, epithelial (adenoma), and mesenchymal (lymphangiomas, lymphangiectasia, neurofibromas, and hemangiomas) neoplasms.[83,84] This section focuses on the lesions that are detectable with VCE and with a known hemorrhagic potential.

- Small bowel lymphangiomas are rare lymphatic system malformations. They are large (2–10 cm) polypoid mucosal based tumors with white-yellowish patches. Approximately one-half of these lesions are associated with anemia or overt GI bleeding, with rare cases of massive bleeding (**Fig. 16**). They are more common in the duodenum and proximal jejunum and can be managed endoscopically, with some requiring surgical resection.[85,86]

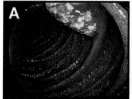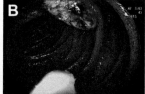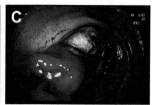

Fig. 16. Bleeding lymphangioma *(spontaneous bleeding, A)* with hemorrhage seen on double balloon enteroscopy with significant hemorrhagic clot with Argon Plasma Coagulation treatment *(B and C).*

- Small bowel hamartomas can be sporadic or related to Peutz–Jeghers polyposis syndrome and juvenile polyposis syndrome. In Peutz–Jeghers polyposis syndrome, multiple hamartomas develop throughout the entire GI tract with a small bowel predilection (prevalence of 70%–96%). Polyp burden ranges from less than 10 to several dozen, with variable morphology and size (diminutive to >4 cm). The juvenile polyposis syndrome prevalence of small bowel polyps is 5% to 14%.[87] Up to 40% of patients with Peutz–Jeghers polyposis syndrome presents with GI bleeding (**Fig. 17**) from ulceration of large polyps. There is a 13% lifetime risk of small bowel cancer and VCE surveillance is recommended.[88]
- Leiomyomas are benign mesenchymal tumors that generally present as small submucosal bulges that are uncommon sources of GI bleeding.
- Brunner's gland hyperplasia is common in the proximal duodenum and seen as multiple diminutive submucosal raised lesions on VCE. Large (>2 cm) Brunner's gland hamartomas can cause IDA, overt GI bleeding, or intermittent obstruction, requiring endoscopic and occasionally surgical intervention.[89]
- Ectopic tissue such as pancreatic heterotopia or gastric heterotopia can present as small bowel (duodenum and jejunum) submucosal lesions.[90] Although predominately asymptomatic in nature, significant bleeding can occur when they are associated with a central mucosal umbilication or ulcer.[91]

Malignant tumors
What are the most common types of small bowel malignancy that lead to gastrointestinal bleeding?
- Adenocarcinomas are most commonly found in the duodenum (50%) and jejunum (20%). Some associated risk factors include celiac disease, familial adenomatous polyposis, and Crohn's disease. VCE findings include protruding masses, ulcerations, strictures, and overt bleeding. The advanced intestinal adenoma precursor to adenocarcinoma can cause mild subacute anemia and rarely overt GI bleeding.[92] Adenocarcinomas often are associated with IDA from ulceration (Video 9) and can present with overt or occult bleeding.

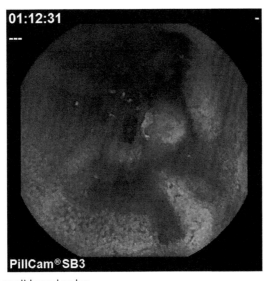

Fig. 17. Bleeding small bowel polyp.

- Neuroendocrine tumors (carcinoids) are typically located in the ileum, including the ileocecal valve (Video 10), and can have multiple synchronous lesions. GI bleeding presentations include mild IDA, occult and overt bleeding, and, uncommonly, massive bleeding (Video 11). VCE imaging includes mass lesion and possible ulcerations overlying a submucosal bulge with surrounding erythematous granular mucosa.[93] The ulceration is often the source of GI bleeding (**Fig. 18**).
- Sarcomas: GI bleeding is common in GI stromal tumors, occurring in 46% in a large case series.[94] VCE typically shows a smooth, round, and protruding submucosal bulging mass with possible central ulceration and associated stigmata of bleeding.[95] Central ulceration or erosions are common and seen in more than one-third of GI stromal tumors and account for the GI bleeding tendency (**Fig. 19**).[88] However, VCE may be limited in characterizing a GI stromal tumor lesion, given the tumor's propensity for extramural growth or localized bleeding obscuring the lesion.[96] GI tract Kaposi sarcoma is a vascular tumor associated with human herpesvirus 8 and seen in about 40% of patients with AIDS. Endoscopic findings are mucosal-based polypoid nodules with a bluish–red complexion that can ulcerate. Patients present with IDA, overt bleeding (including massive bleeding),[97] and bowel obstruction and perforation.[98]
- Primary small bowel lymphomas are mostly B-cell non-Hodgkin's type favoring an ileal (60%) distribution and are commonly associated with bleeding.[99] VCE findings include erythematous thickened mucosa, mucosal plaques, mosaic mucosal pattern (**Fig. 20**), polypoid mass with ulcerations, or nodules.[100]
- Small bowel metastases can occur from a variety of remote primary malignancies (including melanoma, colon, stomach, uterus, ovaries, bladder, breast, lung, and pancreas). Small bowel metastasis can be multifocal and present with IDA or overt GI bleeding. Melanoma has a high small bowel predilection (50% on postmortem examination). Typical lesions are mucosal based and of a blue to deep purple hue, with possible ulcerations (**Fig. 21**).[101]

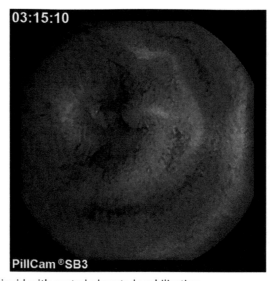

Fig. 18. Ileal carcinoid with central ulcerated umbilication.

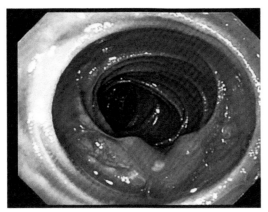

Fig. 19. Ulcerated GI stromal tumor visualized with double balloon enteroscopy.

Video Capsule Endoscopy in Acute and Chronic Gastrointestinal Bleeding

Chronic gastrointestinal bleeding and iron deficiency anemia

Capsule endoscopy is most widely used for nonacute blood loss, because the majority of VCE studies are performed in the outpatient setting. The diagnostic yield of VCE in patients with IDA is approximately 50%,[102–104] with wide ranges as high as 80% in heterogeneous populations and as low as 25.7% in IDA patients without evidence of GI bleeding.[105] One study assessed 620 patients with IDA or occult GI bleeding and reported findings in 33.9% with 68% undergoing further workup and 12.7% requiring therapeutic intervention.[106] Both advancing age and male sex were found to be predictors of definite findings.

In patients less than 50 years of age with IDA, up to one-third had clinically significant small bowel findings, primarily angioectasias and inflammatory lesions. An

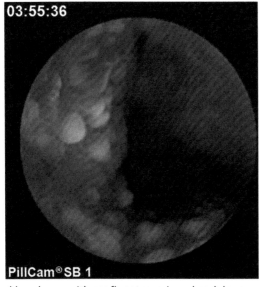

Fig. 20. Small bowel lymphoma with confluent mosaic and nodular mucosa with erythema.

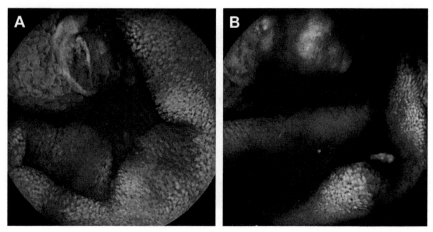

Fig. 21. Metastatic melanoma with ulceration (*A*) and associated bleeding (*B*).

important percentage of diagnoses (5%) however, revealed malignancies,[12] with 1 study showing 25% of those less than 40 years of age with a sinister pathology on VCE, compared with 9% and 0% in the older than 40 and the older than 80 populations, respectively.[107] The overall diagnostic yield tends to be lower in patients less than 50 years of age, but the significant pathology present in some may make VCE use advisable in this group to exclude threatening lesions.[108]

Inpatients with IDA are likely to have higher diagnostic yields of up to 73.4%, given the older age and greater comorbidities. Higher yields have also been associated with increased transit time and nonsteroidal anti-inflammatory drug use.[9] The most common findings (49%) in this cohort were vascular lesions, specifically angioectasias,[106,108] although a variety of other hemorrhagic lesions are potentially detectable in the small bowel as noted elsewhere in this article. One study noted that inpatients with obscure GI bleeding and a negative VCE are unlikely to be readmitted or need intervention during the admission.[109]

The enhanced detection of lesions in patients with IDA was reported with a new capsule technology. Magnetically assisted capsule endoscopy has been used to evaluate patients with recurrent or refractory IDA and was found to detect more total (P<.001) and more IDA associated (P<.04) lesions than EGD. The device was able to provide passive small bowel examination for possible bleeding during the same procedure.[110] The availability of this new technology is limited and will require larger clinical trials.

Acute gastrointestinal bleeding
Acute GI bleeding, determined by hemodynamic stability, rapidity of hemoglobin decrease, and clinical presentation such as melena or hematochezia, is a common cause of hospital admission, with up to 500,000 admissions annually in the United States and mortality rates ranging from 5% to 10%.[1,111] Resuscitation and risk stratification, based on clinical judgment and Blatchford scores, are the cornerstones of initial management. Endoscopic intervention follows in appropriate cases and allows for therapeutics if needed. In these instances, VCE is a second-line diagnostic tool and is not used in the acute setting.

However, the use of capsule technology earlier in the paradigm for acute GI bleeding has occurred. Studies have suggested that the time to endoscopy was shortened if preceded by a positive VCE in the emergency department.[112] A prospective study in emergency department patients discovered that VCE detected upper GI track blood significantly more often than nasogastric tube aspirates in patients with acute GI bleeding.[113] Further studies to explore the role of VCE in rapid diagnostics and triage have followed these initial investigations.

In a study by Schlag and associates,[114] immediately placing a capsule endoscopically in patients with acute severe GI bleeding after a negative EGD resulted in the correct guidance of subsequent therapy in 85% of patients. Another prospective randomized controlled study found that the use of VCE for emergency department triage in patients with GI bleeding could identify low-risk patients and decrease the rate of unnecessary hospital admissions without an effect on the 30-day mortality rate.[115] A parallel randomized controlled superiority trial of patients in the immediate evaluation process, either in the emergency department or directly on admission, determined that use of VCE over the standard of care endoscopy significantly improved the localization of the bleeding site and decreased the time to localization with no difference in direct cost of hospitalization.[116]

A recent review and meta-analysis using EGD as a gold standard showed VCE to have a high sensitivity (0.62–1.00), specificity (0.64–1.00), and accuracy (odds ratio, 12:62; area under the curve of 0.82). Patient comfort was improved, and cost and sedation issues were favorable.[117]

There are, of course, limitations to the standard use of VCE in acute GI bleeding, including preparation adequacy with expedited use, incomplete studies, the uncertainty of timely readings, variability in the level of the reader's expertise, a lack of clarity of lesion identification during active bleeding, and an inability to provide therapeutic intervention. VCE devices that use data storage within the capsule may not be suitable for acute use because of an inability to access the data rapidly or view them in real time.

Lower gastrointestinal bleeding

The standard workup for lower GI bleeding presenting as hematochezia or maroon-colored stool involves an evaluation of the colon and terminal ileum. In rare instances, rapid blood loss from an upper GI source can present as hematochezia and EGD may have a role in this setting.[118] One retrospective study looked at the usefulness of VCE versus EGD in patients with hematochezia after a negative colonoscopy. The study numbers were small, but the work showed that VCE had statistically more findings and led to more therapeutic procedures than EGD.[119] The long-term outcomes were not examined. The detection of Meckel's diverticulum by VCE has been reported in a small case series.[120]

At this time, however, small bowel VCE is not indicated or recommended for the evaluation of hematochezia, although new panendoscopic capsules may detect luminal blood.

Special Populations

Small bowel bleeding in cirrhosis

Cirrhotic patients are at risk for esophagogastric variceal hemorrhage, but can also develop blood loss and IDA from small bowel angioectasias and mucosal oozing associated with portal hypertensive gastropathy and enteropathy. VCE findings include mucosal edema, erythema, a reticulated pattern, erosions, and vascular lesions such as angioectasias and varices.[121,122]

Early VCE studies in cirrhotics reported a 7% to 8% incidence of SBV (**Fig. 22**).[123] A more recent study however, reported a significantly higher presence of SBV in up to 67%.[124] Heightened awareness or more precise imaging may contribute to these disparities.

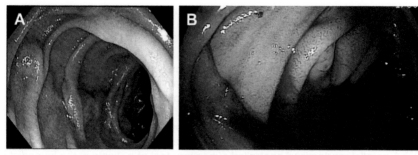

Fig. 22. SBV with bluish serpiginous subepithelial bulge (A) and bleeding (B).

Small bowel bleeding in chronic kidney disease and end-stage renal disease

Initial studies on GI bleeding in patients with chronic kidney disease (CKD) and end-stage renal disease were done before wide availability of VCE. Vascular ectasias are 4 to 10 times more common in patients with CKD than in those with normal kidney function. The duration and severity of the CKD are risk factors for angioectasias.[125] A small prospective study using a first-generation VCE (M2A capsule) showed a prevalence of angioectasias of 47% in patients with CKD. Lesions can be singular or multiple in both the jejunum and ileum.[126] More than one-half of patients with CKD with angioectasias and subsequent blood loss rebleed from the same source.[127] There is a 35% to 40% increased risk for rebleeding after endoscopic therapy in patients with CKD.[128,129]

Small bowel bleeding in patients with a left ventricular assist device

The population of cardiac patients implanted with LVADs has increased dramatically in the last 10 years. The use of VCE in LVAD patients both in the inpatient and outpatient setting has increased accordingly. Between 18% and 40% of patients with a continuous flow LVAD experience GI bleeding after implantation, likely associated with chronic anticoagulation and the nonpulsatile flow state.[130] A pooled analysis noted location of GI bleeding in LVADs to be primarily in the upper GI tract with 48% in the upper GI tract, 15% in the small bowel, 22% in the lower GI tract, and 19% unknown.[131] No confirmed guidelines exist for the assessment of acute bleeding or VCE use in this population and standard endoscopic algorithms typically apply. Decisions are usually made based on expert opinion because there is insufficient evidence for a definitive recommendation.

Given the enhanced morbidity of hospitalized patients an LVAD, many centers aim to limit repeated endoscopic interventions and recommend the first-line use of VCE in patients with an LVAD with melena using-institution specific pathways. Although manufacturer warnings still exist, VCE in this setting is considered safe and studies have documented no interference between the capsule and the implanted device.[132,133] Using VCE in the standard algorithm is the practice, although some investigators have recommended starting directly with VCE for recurrent bleeding in an acute setting, because small bowel lesions are common and most patients have had prior bidirectional endoscopies.

Small bowel bleeding in intensive care patients

Another population in which VCE has a role during episodes of GI bleeding is the patient in the intensive care unit. Patients in the intensive care unit have multiple comorbidities and may tolerate a minimally invasive procedure such as VCE over endoscopic procedures, which present additional risks. Observations of these patients, however, have noted that although lesion detection in this population is high, the usefulness of

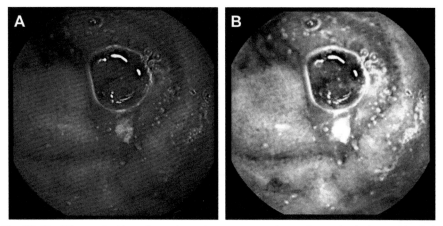

Fig. 23. Flexible spectral imaging color enhancement–enhanced vascular lesion: white light (A), flexible spectral imaging color enhancement 1 (B).

this testing is uncertain, unless patients are prepared to undergo more invasive or surgical procedures.[134] However, the identification of lesions such as metastatic disease or diffuse processes is beneficial if it guides further management.

New Advances and Future Needs

The critical role of VCE in the ability to detect small bowel hemorrhagic lesions has sparked demand for innovations in VCE technology. Prototypes of capsules using legs, paddles, cilia, or vibrations do not approach readiness for clinical use, but devices using external magnets for localization and control show promise for identifying hemorrhagic lesions in the stomach and upper small bowel.[135] Existing software improvements in heme visualization include the suspected blood indicator, QuickView, abnormal lesion detector, and ExpressView. These modalities have not shown superior sensitivity or specificity over conventional viewing.

Narrow band imaging, however, allows for the enhancement of heme-related lesions, and F1 settings on flexible spectral imaging color enhancement amplify the appearance of vascular lesions (**Fig. 23**). Recently, ideas about improving the detection of hemorrhagic VCE lesions using artificial intelligence have emerged. Deep learning techniques and convolutional neural networks seem to be uniquely suited for application in VCE technology.

Strategies have been developed for automatic bleeding detection using VCE dataset images.[136] One CNN algorithm, refined specifically to identify GI angioectasias, yielded a sensitivity for GI angioectasias detection of 100% and specificity of 96% with optimal reproducibility and decreased reading times.[137] Not yet mainstream, these platforms, however, establish a foundation of highly accurate, automated small bowel VCE reading software that will assist in better detection and characterization of lesions causing small bowel bleeding.

SUMMARY

The role of VCE in GI bleeding has long been established in society guidelines as the first-line tool for suspected small bowel bleeding. Aspects of use, such as procedure timing and repeat studies have become clearer yet continue to need clarification. The variety of small bowel hemorrhagic lesions detectable by VCE is robust and incorporates vascular and nonvascular lesions, solitary and systemic, and benign and malignant. This device's role in various populations, such as cirrhotics, inpatients, patients with renal disease, and patients with an LVAD, is confirmed and useful, and its use in acute settings is becoming more frequent and feasible. Innovations to improve the precision of VCE's bleeding detection are growing, particularly in the realm of artificial intelligence. This factor will likely confirm VCE's plasticity and solidify its role in the vanguard of GI bleeding diagnostic technology.

CLINICS CARE POINTS

- VCE is the first-line study for the evaluation of suspected small bowel bleeding and has an increased diagnostic yield if performed within 3 days of a bleeding event.
- Angioectasias are the most common cause of small bowel bleeding found on VCE. In addition, VCE detects a wide range of hemorrhagic mucosal lesions including large vessel abnormalities and nonvascular lesions such as ulcerations, inflammation, and neoplasms.
- The identification of hemorrhagic lesions with the Saurin classification aids in risk stratification and management.
- VCE has an established role in evaluation of IDA and chronic small bowel bleeding, and there is growing evidence that VCE may have a role in acute settings in the ED or in urgent management decisions.
- The use of VCE in the LVAD population is safe and may be used early in the rebleeding evaluation to avoid risks of endoscopy.
- A negative VCE in the setting of GI bleeding evaluation risk stratifies rebleeding to less than 20%.

DISCLOSURE

R.M. Wu – Medtronic Education Grant. L.R. Fisher – Medtronic.

SUPPLEMENTARY DATA

Supplementary data related to this article can be found online at https://doi.org/10.1016/j.giec.2020.12.003.

REFERENCES

1. Peery AF, Crockett SD, Barritt AS, et al. Burden of gastrointestinal, liver, and pancreatic diseases in the United States. Gastroenterology 2015;149(7): 1731–41.e3.
2. Capsule Endoscopy Market Analysis. In: Reports and Data. 2019. Available at: https://www.reportsanddata.com/report-detail/capsule-endoscopy-market. Accessed July 25,2020.
3. Gerson LB, Fidler JL, Cave DR, et al. ACG clinical guideline: diagnosis and management of small bowel bleeding. Am J Gastroenterol 2015;110(9): 1265–87.
4. Gurudu SR, Bruining DH, Acosta RD, et al. The role of endoscopy in the management of suspected small-bowel bleeding. Gastrointest Endosc 2017;85(1): 22–31.

5. Enns RA, Hookey L, Armstrong D, et al. Clinical practice guidelines for the use of video capsule endoscopy. Gastroenterology 2017;152(3):497–514.
6. Rondonotti E, Villa F, Mulder CJ, et al. Small bowel capsule endoscopy in 2007: indications, risks and limitations. World J Gastroenterol 2007;13(46):6140–9.
7. Sealock RJ, Thrift AP, El-Serag HB, et al. Long-term follow up of patients with obscure gas bleeding examined with video capsule endoscopy. Medicine (Baltimore) 2018;97(29):e11429.
8. Fisher L, Lee Krinsky M, Anderson MA, et al. The role of endoscopy in the management of obscure GI bleeding. Gastrointest Endosc 2010;72(3):471–9.
9. Kuo JR, Pasha SF, Leighton JA. The clinician's guide to suspected small bowel bleeding. Am J Gastroenterol 2019;114(4):591–8.
10. Hakimian S, Patel K, Cave D. Sending in the ViCE squad: evaluation and management of patients with small intestinal bleeding. Dig Dis Sci 2020;65(5): 1307–14.
11. Van de Bruaene C, Hindryckx P, Snauwaert C, et al. The predictive value of negative capsule endoscopy for the indication of Obscure Gastrointestinal Bleeding: no reassurance in the long term. Acta Gastroenterol Belg 2016; 79(4):405–13.
12. Yung DE, Koulaouzidis A, Avni T, et al. Clinical outcomes of negative small-bowel capsule endoscopy for small-bowel bleeding: a systematic review and meta-analysis. Gastrointest Endosc 2017;85(2):305–17.e2, 7.
13. Macdonald J, Porter V, McNamara D. Negative capsule endoscopy in patients with obscure GI bleeding predicts low rebleeding rates. Gastrointest Endosc 2008;68(6):1122–7.
14. Elijah D, Daas A, Brady P. Capsule endoscopy for obscure GI bleeding yields a high incidence of significant treatable lesions within reach of standard upper endoscopy. J Clin Gastroenterol 2008;42(8):962–3.
15. Viazis N, Papaxoinis K, Vlachogiannakos J, et al. Is there a role for second-look capsule endoscopy in patients with obscure GI bleeding after a nondiagnostic first test? Gastrointest Endosc 2009;69(4):850–6.
16. Wetwittayakhlang P, Wonglhow J, Netinatsunton N, et al. Re-bleeding and its predictors after capsule endoscopy in patients with obscure gastrointestinal bleeding in long-term follow-up. BMC Gastroenterol 2019;19(1):216.
17. Harada A, Torisu T, Okamoto Y, et al. Predictive factors for rebleeding after negative capsule endoscopy among patients with overt obscure gastrointestinal bleeding. Digestion 2020;101(2):129–36.
18. Singh A, Marshall C, Chaudhuri B, et al. Timing of video capsule endoscopy relative to overt obscure GI bleeding: implications from a retrospective study. Gastrointest Endosc 2013;77(5):761–6.
19. Katsinelos P, Chatzimavroudis G, Terzoudis S, et al. Diagnostic yield and clinical impact of capsule endoscopy in obscure gastrointestinal bleeding during routine clinical practice: a single-center experience. Med Princ Pract 2011; 20(1):60–5.
20. Bresci G, Parisi G, Bertoni M, et al. The role of video capsule endoscopy for evaluating obscure gastrointestinal bleeding: usefulness of early use. J Gastroenterol 2005;40(3):256–9.
21. Apostolopoulos P, Liatsos C, Gralnek IM, et al. Evaluation of capsule endoscopy in active, mild-to moderate, overt, obscure GI bleeding. Gastrointest Endosc 2007;66(6):1174–81.
22. Rondonotti E, Spada C, Adler S, et al. Small-bowel capsule endoscopy and device-assisted enteroscopy for diagnosis and treatment of small-bowel

disorders: European Society of Gastrointestinal Endoscopy (ESGE) Technical Review. Endoscopy 2018;50(4):423–46.

23. Liao Z, Gao R, Xu C, et al. Indications and detection, completion, and retention rates of small-bowel capsule endoscopy: a systematic review. Gastrointest Endosc 2010;71(2):280–6.

24. Song JH, Hong SN, Kyung Chang D, et al. The etiology of potential small-bowel bleeding depending on patient's age and gender. United Eur Gastroenterol J 2018;6(8):1169–78.

25. Pasha SF, Leighton JA. Evidence-based guide on capsule endoscopy for small bowel bleeding. Gastroenterol Hepatol (N Y) 2017;13(2):88–93.

26. Sidhu R, Sanders DS, Kapur K, et al. Factors predicting the diagnostic yield and intervention in obscure gastrointestinal bleeding investigated using capsule endoscopy. J Gastrointestin Liver Dis 2009;18(3):273–8.

27. Saurin JC, Delvaux M, Gaudin JL, et al. Diagnostic value of endoscopic capsule in patients with obscure digestive bleeding: blinded comparison with video push-enteroscopy. Endoscopy 2003;35(7):576–84.

28. Becq A, Rahmi G, Perrod G, et al. Hemorrhagic angiodysplasia of the digestive tract: pathogenesis, diagnosis, and management. Gastrointest Endosc 2017; 86(5):792–806.

29. Yano T, Yamamoto H, Sunada K, et al. Endoscopic classification of vascular lesions of the small intestine (with videos). Gastrointest Endosc 2008;67(1): 169–72.

30. García-Compeán D, Del Cueto-Aguilera ÁN, Jiménez-Rodríguez AR, et al. Diagnostic and therapeutic challenges of gastrointestinal angiodysplasias: a critical review and view points. World J Gastroenterol 2019;25(21):2549–64.

31. Saurin JC, Jacob P, Pioche M. Treatment of digestive angioectasia: time for prospective, randomized, therapeutic studies. Endosc Int Open 2019;7(12): E1778–9.

32. Boal Carvalho P, Magalhães J, Dias de Castro F, et al. Virtual chromoendoscopy improves the diagnostic yield of small bowel capsule endoscopy in obscure gastrointestinal bleeding. Dig Liver Dis 2016;48(2):172–5.

33. Maeda M, Hiraishi H. Efficacy of video capsule endoscopy with flexible spectral imaging color enhancement at setting 3 for differential diagnosis of red spots in the small bowel. Dig Endosc 2014;26(2):228–31.

34. Jackson CS, Strong R. Gastrointestinal angiodysplasia: diagnosis and management. Gastrointest Endosc Clin N Am 2017;27(1):51–62.

35. Douard R, Wind P, Berger A, et al. Role of intraoperative enteroscopy in the management of obscure gastrointestinal bleeding at the time of video-capsule endoscopy. Am J Surg 2009;198(1):6–11.

36. Jackson CS, Gerson LB. Management of gastrointestinal angiodysplastic lesions (GIADs): a systematic review and meta-analysis. Am J Gastroenterol 2014;109(4):474–84.

37. Heyde EC. Gastrointestinal bleeding in aortic stenosis [letter]. N Engl J Med 1958;259:196.

38. Vincentelli A, Susen S, Le Tourneau T, et al. Acquired von Willebrand syndrome in aortic stenosis. N Engl J Med 2003;349(4):343–9, 1.

39. Thompson JL, Schaff AV, Dearani JA, et al. Risk of recurrent gastrointestinal bleeding after aortic valve replacement in patients with Heyde syndrome. J Thorac Cardiovasc Surg 2012;144(1):112–6.

40. Tachecí I, Bradna P, Douda T, et al. NSAID-induced enteropathy in rheumatoid arthritis patients with chronic occult gastrointestinal bleeding: a prospective capsule endoscopy study. Gastroenterol Res Pract 2013;2013:268382.

41. Grève E, Moussata D, Gaudin JL, et al. High diagnostic and clinical impact of small-bowel capsule endoscopy in patients with hereditary hemorrhagic telangiectasia with overt digestive bleeding and/or severe anemia. Gastrointest Endosc 2010;71(4):760–7.

42. Singh K, Zubair A, Prindle A, et al. Diagnostic yield of capsule endoscopy for small bowel arteriovenous malformations in patients with hereditary hemorrhagic telangiectasia: a systematic review and meta-analysis. Endosc Int Open 2019;7(2):E282–9.

43. Wang ZK, Wang FY, Zhu RM, et al. Klippel-Trenaunay syndrome with gastrointestinal bleeding, splenic hemangiomas and left inferior vena cava. World J Gastroenterol 2010;16(12):1548–52.

44. Maeda Y, Moribata K, Deguchi H, et al. Video capsule endoscopy as the initial examination for overt obscure gastrointestinal bleeding can efficiently identify patients who require double-balloon enteroscopy. BMC Gastroenterol 2015; 15:132.

45. de Franchis R, Rondonotti E, Abbiati C, et al. Successful identification of a jejunal Dieulafoy lesion by wireless capsule enteroscopy: a case report. Dig Liver Dis 2002;34:A118.

46. Dulic-Lakovic E, Dulic M, Hubner D, et al. Bleeding Dieulafoy lesions of the small bowel: a systematic study on the epidemiology and efficacy of enteroscopic treatment. Gastrointest Endosc 2011;74(3):573–80.

47. Tang SJ, Zanati S, Dubcenco E, et al. Diagnosis of small-bowel varices by capsule endoscopy. Gastrointest Endosc 2004;60(1):129–35.

48. Barlas A, Avsar E, Bozbas A, et al. Role of capsule endoscopy in blue rubber bleb nevus syndrome. Can J Surg 2008;51(6):E119–20.

49. Isoldi S, Belsha D, Yeop I, et al. Diagnosis and management of children with blue rubber bleb nevus syndrome: a multi-center case series. Dig Liver Dis 2019;51(11):1537–46.

50. Akhrass R, Yaffe MB, Fischer C, et al. Small-bowel diverticulosis: perceptions and reality. J Am Coll Surg 1997;184:383–8.

51. Baltes P, Matsui U, Sievers J, et al. Jejunal diverticulum with active bleeding. Video J Encyclopedia GI Endosc 2013;1:248–9.

52. Sagar J, Kumar V, Shah DK. Meckel's diverticulum: a systematic review [published correction appears in J R Soc Med. 2007 Feb;100(2):69]. J R Soc Med 2006;99(10):501–5.

53. Dubcenco E, Tang SJ, Streutker CJ, et al. Meckel's diverticulum mimicking small bowel tumor. Gastrointest Endosc 2004;60:263.

54. Kida A, Matsuda K, Hirai S, et al. A pedunculated polyp-shaped small-bowel lymphangioma causing gastrointestinal bleeding and treated by double-balloon enteroscopy. World J Gastroenterol 2012;18(34):4798–800.

55. Herfarth H, Hofstädter F, Feuerbach S, et al. A case of recurrent gastrointestinal bleeding and protein-losing gastroenteropathy. Nat Rev Gastroenterol Hepatol 2007;4:288–93.

56. Huang MY, Chang HM, Gao HW, et al. Small intestinal lymphangioma with lymphangioectasia causing obscure gastrointestinal bleeding. Am J Gastroenterol 2017;112(3):413.

57. Wiedbrauck F. Benign Tumors. In: Keuchel M, Hagenmuller F, H Tajiri M, editors. Video capsule endoscopy. A reference guide and Atlas. Berlin: Springer; 2014. p. 317–36.

58. James DG, Zuckerman GR, Sayuk GS, et al. Clinical recognition of AI type amyloidosis of the luminal gastrointestinal tract. Clin Gastroenterol Hepatol 2007;5(5):582–8.

59. Guagnozzi D, Lucendo AJ. Anemia in inflammatory bowel disease: a neglected issue with relevant effects. World J Gastroenterol 2014;20(13):3542–51.

60. Melmed GY, Dubinsky MC, Rubin DT, et al. Utility of video capsule endoscopy for longitudinal monitoring of Crohn's disease activity in the small bowel: a prospective study. Gastrointest Endosc 2018;88(6):947–55.e2.

61. Flamant M, Trang C, Maillard O, et al. The prevalence and outcome of jejunal lesions visualized by small bowel capsule endoscopy in Crohn's disease. Inflamm Bowel Dis 2013;19(7):1390–6.

62. Bojesen RD, Riis LB, Høgdall E, et al. Inflammatory bowel disease and small bowel cancer risk, clinical characteristics, and histopathology: a population-based study. Clin Gastroenterol Hepatol 2017;15(12):1900–7.e2.

63. Podugu A, Tandon K, Castro FJ. Crohn's disease presenting as acute gastrointestinal hemorrhage. World J Gastroenterol 2016;22(16):4073–8.

64. Pardi DS, Loftus EV Jr, Tremaine WJ, et al. Acute major gastrointestinal hemorrhage in inflammatory bowel disease. Gastrointest Endosc 1999;49(2):153–7.

65. Collin P, Rondonotti E, Lundin KE, et al. Video capsule endoscopy in celiac disease: current clinical practice. J Dig Dis 2012;13(2):94–9.

66. Nehra V. New clinical issues in celiac disease. Gastroenterol Clin North Am 1998;27(2):453–65.

67. Goldstein JL, Eisen GM, Lewis B, et al. Video capsule endoscopy to prospectively assess small bowel injury with celecoxib, naproxen plus omeprazole, and placebo. Clin Gastroenterol Hepatol 2005;3(2):133–41.

68. Maiden L, Thjodleifsson B, Theodors A, et al. A quantitative analysis of NSAID-induced small bowel pathology by capsule enteroscopy. Gastroenterology 2005;128(5):1172–8.

69. Lang J, Price AB, Levi AJ, et al. Diaphragm disease: pathology of disease of the small intestine induced by non-steroidal anti-inflammatory drugs. J Clin Pathol 1988;41(5):516–26.

70. Arimoto J, Endo H, Kato T, et al. Clinical value of capsule endoscopy for detecting small bowel lesions in patients with intestinal Behçet's disease. Dig Endosc 2016;28(2):179–85.

71. Hisamatsu T, Naganuma M, Matsuoka K, et al. Diagnosis and management of intestinal Behçet's disease. Clin J Gastroenterol 2014;7(3):205–12.

72. Pulimood AB, Amarapurkar DN, Ghoshal U, et al. Differentiation of Crohn's disease from intestinal tuberculosis in India in 2010. World J Gastroenterol 2011; 17(4):433–43.

73. Debi U, Ravisankar V, Prasad KK, et al. Abdominal tuberculosis of the gastrointestinal tract: revisited. World J Gastroenterol 2014;20(40):14831–40.

74. Kela M, Agrawal A, Sharma R, et al. Ileal tuberculosis presenting as a case of massive rectal bleeding. Clin Exp Gastroenterol 2009;2:129–31.

75. National Cancer Institute. Cancer stat facts: small intestine cancer. Available at: https://seer.cancer.gov/statfacts/html/smint.html. Accessed July 25,2020.

76. Rondonotti E, Pennazio M, Toth E, et al. Small-bowel neoplasms in patients undergoing video capsule endoscopy: a multicenter European study. Endoscopy 2008;40:488–95.

77. Lewis BS, Kornbluth A, Waye JD. Small bowel tumours: yield of enteroscopy. Gut 1991;32(7):763–5.
78. Lewis BS, Eisen GM, Friedman S. A pooled analysis to evaluate results of capsule endoscopy trials. Endoscopy 2005;37(10):960–5 [erratum appears in Endoscopy. 2007 Mar;39(4):303].
79. Cobrin GM, Pittman RH, Lewis BS. Increased diagnostic yield of small bowel tumors with capsule endoscopy. Cancer 2006;107:22–7.
80. Girelli CM, Porta P, Colombo E, et al. Development of a novel index to discriminate bulge from mass on small-bowel capsule endoscopy. Gastrointest Endosc 2011;74(5):1067–115.e5.
81. Min M, Noujaim M, Green J, et al. Role of mucosal protrusion angle in discriminating between true and false masses of the small bowel on video capsule endoscopy. J Clin Med 2019;8(4) [pii:E418].
82. Saito H, Aoki T, Aoyama K, et al. Automatic detection and classification of protruding lesions in wireless capsule endoscopy images based on a deep convolutional neural network. Gastrointest Endosc 2020;92(1):144–51.e1.
83. de Latour RA, Kilaru SM, Gross SA. Management of small bowel polyps: a literature review. Best Pract Res Clin Gastroenterol 2017;31(4):401–8.
84. Cheung DY, Lee IS, Chang DK, et al. Capsule endoscopy in small bowel tumors: a multicenter Korean study. J Gastroenterol Hepatol 2010;25(6):1079–86.
85. Xiao NJ, Ning SB, Li T, et al. Small intestinal hemolymphangioma treated with enteroscopic injection sclerotherapy: a case report and review of literature. World J Gastroenterol 2020;26(13):1540–5.
86. Tang SJ, Bhaijee Feriyl. Small bowel lymphangioma. Video J Encyclopedia GI Endosc 2014;1(3–4):663–5.
87. Gilad O, Rosner G, Fliss-Isakov N, et al. Clinical and histologic overlap and distinction among various hamartomatous polyposis syndromes. Clin Transl Gastroenterol 2019;10(5):1–9.
88. Syngal S, Brand RE, Church JM, et al. ACG clinical guideline: genetic testing and management of hereditary gastrointestinal cancer syndromes. Am J Gastroenterol 2015;110(2):223–63.
89. Frenkel NC, Laclé MM, Borel Rinkes IH, et al. A giant brunneroma causing gastrointestinal bleeding and severe anemia requiring transfusion and surgery. Case Rep Surg 2017;2017:6940649.
90. Chen HL, Lin SC, Chang WH, et al. Identification of ectopic pancreas in the ileum by capsule endoscopy. J Formos Med Assoc 2007;106(3):240–3.
91. Lee MJ, Chang JH, Maeng IH, et al. Ectopic pancreas bleeding in the jejunum revealed by capsule endoscopy. Clin Endosc 2012;45(3):194–7.
92. Singh KL, Prabhu T, Gunjiganvi M, et al. Isolated duodenal adenoma presenting as gastrointestinal bleed - a case report. J Clin Diagn Res 2014;8(6):ND01–2.
93. Gustafsson BI, Siddique L, Chan A, et al. Uncommon cancers of the small intestine, appendix and colon: an analysis of SEER 1973-2004, and current diagnosis and therapy. Int J Oncol 2008;33(6):1121–31.
94. Zhou L, Liao Y, Wu J, et al. Small bowel gastrointestinal stromal tumor: a retrospective study of 32 cases at a single center and review of the literature. Ther Clin Risk Manag 2018;14:1467–81.
95. Kauser R, Kazemi A, Farah K, et al. Easy to swallow: detection of an extramural jejunal GIST by video capsule endoscopy. BMJ Case Rep 2015;2015. bcr2015211192.
96. Gaspar JP, Stelow EB, Wang AY. Approach to the endoscopic resection of duodenal lesions. World J Gastroenterol 2016;22(2):600–17.

97. Neville CR, Peddada AV, Smith D, et al. Massive gastrointestinal hemorrhage from AIDS-related Kaposi's sarcoma confined to the small bowel managed with radiation. Med Pediatr Oncol 1996;26(2):135–8.

98. Arora M, Goldberg EM. Kaposi sarcoma involving the gastrointestinal tract. Gastroenterol Hepatol (N Y) 2010;6(7):459–62.

99. Ghimire P, Wu GY, Zhu L. Primary gastrointestinal lymphoma. World J Gastroenterol 2011;17(6):697–707.

100. Flieger D, Keller R, May A, et al. Capsule endoscopy in gastrointestinal lymphomas. Endoscopy 2005;37(12):1174–80.

101. Lewis BS. Malignant tumors. In: Keuchel M, Hagenmuller F, editors. Video capsule endoscopy. Springer; 2014. p. 337–58.

102. Koulaouzidis A, Rondonotti E, Giannakou A, et al. Diagnostic yield of small-bowel capsule endoscopy in patients with iron-deficiency anemia: a systematic review. Gastrointest Endosc 2012;76(5):983–92.

103. Olano C, Pazos X, Avendaño K, et al. Diagnostic yield and predictive factors of findings in small-bowel capsule endoscopy in the setting of iron-deficiency anemia. Endosc Int Open 2018;6(6):E688–93.

104. Xavier S, Magalhães J, Rosa B, et al. Impact of small bowel capsule endoscopy in iron deficiency anemia: influence of patient's age on diagnostic yield. Arq Gastroenterol 2018;55(3):242–6.

105. Tong J, Svarta S, Ou G, et al. Diagnostic yield of capsule endoscopy in the setting of iron deficiency anemia without evidence of gastrointestinal bleeding. Can J Gastroenterol 2012;26(10):687–90.

106. Stone J, Grover K, Bernstein CN. The use of capsule endoscopy for diagnosis of iron deficiency anemia: a retrospective analysis. J Clin Gastroenterol 2020; 54(5):452–8.

107. Koulaouzidis A, Yung DE, Lam JH, et al. The use of small-bowel capsule endoscopy in iron-deficiency anemia alone; be aware of the young anemic patient. Scand J Gastroenterol 2012;47(8–9):1094–100.

108. Sidhu PS, McAlindon ME, Drew K, et al. The utility of capsule endoscopy in patients under 50 years of age with recurrent iron deficiency anaemia: is the juice worth the squeeze? Gastroenterol Res Pract 2015;2015:948574.

109. Alsahafi M, Cramer P, Chatur N, et al. The impact of inpatient capsule endoscopy on the need for therapeutic interventions in patients with obscure gastrointestinal bleeding. Saudi J Gastroenterol 2020;26(1):53–60.

110. Ching HL, Hale MF, Sidhu R, et al. Magnetically assisted capsule endoscopy in suspected acute upper GI bleeding versus esophagogastroduodenoscopy in detecting focal lesions. Gastrointest Endosc 2019;90(3):430–9.

111. Loperfido S, Baldo V, Piovesana E, et al. Changing trends in acute upper-GI bleeding: a population-based study. Gastrointest Endosc 2009;70(2):212–24.

112. Rubin M, Hussain SA, Shalomov A, et al. Live view video capsule endoscopy enables risk stratification of patients with acute upper GI bleeding in the emergency room: a pilot study. Dig Dis Sci 2011;56(3):786–91.

113. Gralnek IM, Ching JY, Maza I, et al. Capsule endoscopy in acute upper gastrointestinal hemorrhage: a prospective cohort study. Endoscopy 2013;45(1):12–9.

114. Schlag C, Menzel C, Nennstiel S, et al. Emergency video capsule endoscopy in patients with acute severe GI bleeding and negative upper endoscopy results. Gastrointest Endosc 2015;81(4):889–95.

115. Sung JJ, Tang RS, Ching JY, et al. Use of capsule endoscopy in the emergency department as a triage of patients with GI bleeding. Gastrointest Endosc 2016; 84(6):907–13.

116. Marya NB, Jawaid S, Foley A, et al. A randomized controlled trial comparing efficacy of early video capsule endoscopy with standard of care in the approach to nonhematemesis GI bleeding (with videos). Gastrointest Endosc 2019;89(1): 33–43.e34.
117. Shah N, Chen C, Montano N, et al. Video capsule endoscopy for upper gastrointestinal hemorrhage in the emergency department: a systematic review and meta-analysis. Am J Emerg Med 2020;38(6):1245–52.
118. Kamboj AK, Hoversten P, Leggett CL. Upper gastrointestinal bleeding: etiologies and management. Mayo Clin Proc 2019;94(4):697–703, 2.
119. Aoki T, Nagata N, Yamada A, et al. Next endoscopic approach for acute lower gastrointestinal bleeding without an identified source on colonoscopy: upper or capsule endoscopy? Endosc Int Open 2019;7(3):E337–46.
120. Lin L, Liu K, Liu H, et al. Capsule endoscopy as a diagnostic test for Meckel's diverticulum. Scand J Gastroenterol 2019;54(1):122–7.
121. Tavakkoli A, Spencer M, Takami M, et al. Video of the month: actively bleeding idiopathic vascular bleb found via double-balloon enteroscopy. Am J Gastroenterol 2015;110(1):16.
122. Aoyama T, Oka S, Aikata H, et al. Small bowel abnormalities in patients with compensated liver cirrhosis. Dig Dis Sci 2013;58(5):1390–6.
123. De Palma GD, Rega M, Masone S, et al. Mucosal abnormalities of the small bowel in patients with cirrhosis and portal hypertension: a capsule endoscopy study. Gastrointest Endosc 2005;62(4):529–34.
124. Goenka MK, Shah BB, Rai VK, et al. Mucosal changes in the small intestines in portal hypertension: first study using the pillcam SB3 capsule endoscopy system. Clin Endosc 2018;51(6):563–9.
125. Chalasani N, Cotsonis G, Wilcox CM. Upper gastrointestinal bleeding in patients with chronic renal failure: role of vascular ectasia. Am J Gastroenterol 1996; 91(11):2329–32.
126. Karagiannis S, Goulas S, Kosmadakis G, et al. Wireless capsule endoscopy in the investigation of patients with chronic renal failure and obscure gastrointestinal bleeding (preliminary data). World J Gastroenterol 2006;12(32):5182–5.
127. Zuckerman GR, Cornette GL, Clouse RE, et al. Upper gastrointestinal bleeding in patients with chronic renal failure. Ann Intern Med 1985;102(5):588–92.
128. Pinho R, Ponte A, Rodrigues A, et al. Long-term rebleeding risk following endoscopic therapy of small-bowel vascular lesions with device-assisted enteroscopy. Eur J Gastroenterol Hepatol 2016;28(4):479–85.
129. Romagnuolo J, Brock AS, Ranney N. Is Endoscopic therapy effective for angioectasia in obscure gastrointestinal bleeding? A systematic review of the literature. J Clin Gastroenterol 2015;49(10):823–30.
130. Molina TL, Krisl JC, Donahue KR, et al. Gastrointestinal bleeding in left ventricular assist device: octreotide and other treatment modalities. Asaio j 2018;64(4): 433–9.
131. Draper KV, Huang RJ, Gerson LB. GI bleeding in patients with continuous-flow left ventricular assist devices: a systematic review and meta-analysis. Gastrointest Endosc 2014;80(3):435–46.e1.
132. Tabet R, Nassani N, Karam B, et al. Pooled Analysis of the Efficacy and Safety of Video Capsule Endoscopy in Patients with Implantable Cardiac Devices. Can J Gastroenterol Hepatol 2019;2019:3953807.
133. Harris LA, Hansel SL, Rajan E, et al. Capsule endoscopy in patients with implantable electromedical devices is safe. Gastroenterol Res Pract 2013; 2013:959234.

134. Boutros J, Leblanc S, Pène F. Small-bowel capsule endoscopy for obscure gastrointestinal bleeding in the ICU. Intensive Care Med 2019;45(2):295-8.

135. Rahman I, Pioche M, Shim CS, et al. Magnetic-assisted capsule endoscopy in the upper GI tract by using a novel navigation system (with video). Gastrointest Endosc 2016;83(5):889-95.e1.

136. Xing X, Jia X, Meng MQ. Bleeding detection in wireless capsule endoscopy image video using superpixel-color histogram and a subspace KNN classifier. Conf Proc IEEE Eng Med Biol Soc 2018;2018:1-4.

137. Leenhardt R, Vasseur P, Li C, et al. A neural network algorithm for detection of GI angioectasia during small-bowel capsule endoscopy. Gastrointest Endosc 2019;89(1):189-94.

Timing and Use of Capsule Endoscopy in the Acute Care Setting

Mark Hanscom, MD*, Anupam Singh, MD

KEYWORDS

- Video capsule endoscopy • Acute care setting • Emergency department
- Gastrointestinal bleeding • Chest pain

KEY POINTS

- Early deployment of video capsule endoscopy (VCE) in patients with gastrointestinal bleeding is critical in improving diagnostic yield.
- Data are accumulating for the use of VCE as a first-line diagnostic modality in the evaluation of both hematemesis and nonhematemesis gastrointestinal bleeding.
- VCE might be in particularly useful in the evaluation and triage of patients with gastrointestinal bleeding in resource-limited settings, such as during a pandemic or during weekends.
- PillCam ESO in the evaluation of patients with noncardiac chest pain in the emergency department is both well tolerated and effective in the detection of esophagitis.

INTRODUCTION

Since its introduction in the United States in 2001, the role of video capsule endoscopy (VCE) has continued to evolve. It has demonstrated use in the evaluation of a wide range of gastrointestinal conditions, including inflammatory bowel disease (IBD), small bowel tumors, malabsorptive diseases, and chest pain. However, its most common use is in the evaluation and management of gastrointestinal bleeding that originates in the small intestine.

VIDEO CAPSULE ENDOSCOPY IN SMALL INTESTINAL BLEEDING

In the current algorithmic approach to small intestinal bleeding, VCE remains a second-line procedure behind both upper endoscopy and colonoscopy. In patients presenting with signs of gastrointestinal bleeding, the initial focus should be on immediate assessment and appropriate resuscitation. Current guidelines recommend initial resuscitation with intravascular volume replacement to correct hemodynamic

Division of Gastroenterology, University of Massachusetts Medical School, Memorial Medical Center, 55 Lake Avenue, North Worcester, MA 01650, USA
* Corresponding author.
E-mail address: mark.hanscom@umassmemorial.org

Gastrointest Endoscopy Clin N Am 31 (2021) 307–316
https://doi.org/10.1016/j.giec.2020.12.006
1052-5157/21/© 2020 Elsevier Inc. All rights reserved.

instability, with the goal of normalization of blood pressure and heart rate before endoscopic intervention. In cases with severe anemia, a restrictive red blood cell transfusion strategy should be pursued targeting a hemoglobin greater than 7 g/dL, with higher hemoglobin levels targeted in patients with significant comorbidities, such as coronary artery disease. Pharmacologic treatment is often initiated with a proton-pump inhibitor in bolus or infusion form, and baseline coagulopathies are corrected. Following adequate resuscitation, conventional endoscopy is the standard of care, with upper endoscopy being the test of choice in all cases except for certain lower gastrointestinal bleeding, in which case colonoscopy is warranted.[1–4] In patients who undergo bidirectional conventional endoscopy without identification of a source of bleeding, the diagnosis of obscure gastrointestinal bleeding (OGIB) can then be made. Most of these patients are not further investigated and, fortunately, most do not rebleed. However, these patients are nonetheless left in the unsatisfactory situation of having the source of bleeding remain unknown. If bleeding continues, then some patients will go on to undergo VCE, with 5% to 10% ultimately being diagnosed with small bowel bleeding. This, in all likelihood, underrepresents the true proportion of patients with small bowel bleeding, as many patients will go undiagnosed because bleeding has ceased and thus the source of bleeding cannot be identified. Those patients who do have bleeding from a source within the small intestine are better labeled as having "suspected small intestinal bleeding," with the term OGIB reserved for patients with a negative small bowel evaluation.[5]

The role of VCE in this population of patients with suspected small intestinal bleeding is well-established, with current guidelines recommending VCE as a first-line procedure for small bowel bleeding after upper and lower endoscopy have been performed.[5] In the acute setting, small bowel bleeding can present in a multitude of manners, including melena and hematochezia. Iron-deficiency anemia and guaiac-positive stools reflect a more chronic condition. Overt small bowel bleeding comprises patients presenting with hematochezia or melena after a negative bidirectional endoscopic evaluation, whereas occult small intestinal bleeding comprises patients presenting with a positive fecal occult blood test (with or without iron-deficiency anemia) after a similarly negative endoscopic evaluation. Overall, small bowel sources comprise 5% to 10% of identified lesions in patients presenting with gastrointestinal bleeding.[6] The etiologies of bleeding varies based on age. In patients younger than 40 years, common causes include IBD, Dieulafoy lesions, and neoplasia. In patients older than 40 years, IBD is seen less often, and more common causes include angioectasias, Dieulafoy lesions, and also neoplasia.[5,7]

In cases of suspected small intestinal bleeding, VCE is able to evaluate the entire small bowel in 79% to 90% of cases, with both a high positive (94%–97%) and negative predictive value (83%–100%).[8–10] The overall diagnostic yield of VCE in patients with suspected small intestinal bleeding is 38% to 83%, with higher rates in overt small intestinal bleeding (60%) than in occult small intestinal bleeding (46)%.[11] Other factors that influence diagnostic yield include hemoglobin level, duration of bleeding, timing to acute bleeding episode, male sex, age older than 60 years, and inpatient status.[12–14] Overall, in 37% to 87% of patients, the use of VCE leads to endoscopic intervention or a change in medical management.[10,15] Even in cases in which a bleeding lesion is not identified, VCE offers helpful prognostic information. The rate of rebleeding is significantly lower in patients with a negative capsule study, ranging from 6% to 27%.[16–18] It is, expectedly, higher in patients on anticoagulation.[19] The negative predictive value of VCE in predicting rebleeding can reach as high as 94.4%.[18] Repeat VCE also can be helpful, and should be considered, in patients with a change in presentation from occult to overt bleeding, or with a new hemoglobin drop greater than 4 g/dL.[20] Repeat

VCE can reveal positive findings in up to 35% to 49% of patients. In one small trial, repeat VCE led to a change in clinical management in 10% of cases.[20] Before VCE, patients should be counseled on the rare risk of complications. Although uncommon, complications occur in up to 2% of cases, and include an inability to swallow the capsule, capsule retention, impaction at the cricopharyngeal junction, and rarely aspiration. Most cases of capsule retention are asymptomatic but require elective enteroscopic retrieval or partial small bowel resection for capsule collection and treatment of the underlying cause of retention. The most common cause of capsule retention is Crohn's disease (in which retention can reach up to 13%), followed by nonsteroidal anti-inflammatory drug enteropathy, radiation enteritis, and then obstructive lesions such as carcinoid or metastatic cancer.[21,22] Fortunately, surgical resection of retained capsules is safe and comes with the added benefit of treating the obstructing lesion. More serious complications, such as perforation, are exceedingly rare.[23]

VCE offers clear advantages compared with other diagnostic modalities in the overt bleeding setting. To date, studies have demonstrated improved diagnostic yield with VCE when compared with angiography, barium radiography, and push enteroscopy in the evaluation of small bowel bleeding. For example, in cases of overt small intestinal bleeding, immediate VCE improved diagnostic yield compared with angiography (53% vs 20%) without significant differences in transfusion requirements, admissions for rebleeding, or mortality.[24] In another prospective evaluation of patients with OGIB, VCE was able to detect a source of bleeding in more patients (72%) than either computed tomography angiography (24%) or standard mesenteric angiography (56%).[25] VCE also holds an advantage over push enteroscopy in terms of both detecting bleeding lesions and affecting clinical certainty, without sacrificing changes in rebleeding rates or resource utilization up to 12 months after testing. In a large meta-analysis comparing the yield of different diagnostic modalities in cases of small intestinal bleeding, the yield of VCE was superior to both barium radiography (67% vs 8%) and push enteroscopy (63% vs 28%). The number-needed-to-test with VCE to establish 1 additional clinically significant finding over either barium radiography or push enteroscopy was 3. Most of this incremental yield came from the improved visualization of flat vascular and small inflammatory lesions.[26] Given its high diagnostic yield, VCE is therefore the test of choice in the evaluation of small bowel bleeding after unrevealing conventional endoscopy.

VCE also should be considered before therapeutic intervention. The use of preprocedural VCE to "map" the small bowel has been demonstrated to improve clinical outcomes and increase the proportion of patients receiving therapeutic intervention. For example, in one trial that coordinated preprocedural VCE with intraoperative enteroscopy (IOE) in 18 patients, IOE resulted in treatment in 87% of patients with a prior positive VCE, compared with 0% of patients with a prior negative VCE. This suggests an important directive role of VCE in optimizing therapeutic interventions.[27]

TIMING OF CAPSULE ENDOSCOPY

Gastrointestinal bleeding, when not severe, can be fleeting and difficult to diagnose. Overall, in 80% of cases, gastrointestinal bleeding will stop on its own. The remaining 20% of cases that do not self-resolve will require some level of support and intervention. Of those cases that do stop spontaneously, a significant but unknown proportion will have ceased bleeding by the time of presentation. Some of these patients will go undiagnosed as to the source of bleeding, whereas others will have bleeding attributed to coexistent lesions, which may or may not have been the culprit source of bleeding. This "endoscopic rationalization" can result in very different data on the sources of bleeding when compared with data from detection of active bleeding or lesions with stigmata of recent hemorrhage, thereby altering our understanding of the epidemiology of gastrointestinal bleeding.

In the current clinical environment, VCE is a second-line test, often performed far out from the initial presentation after endoscopy, colonoscopy, and perhaps other endoscopic or radiographic modalities have been exhausted. However, more and more studies suggest that when it comes to VCE, the earlier it is performed the better. The European Society of Gastrointestinal Endoscopy (ESGE), for instance, recommends VCE "as soon as possible after the bleeding episode, optimally within 14-days, in order to maximize the diagnostic yield."[28] The advantages of earlier timing of VCE are numerous, and as capsule technologies continue to evolve, serious consideration should be given to immediate VCE in the emergency department (ED) and other acute settings.

To start, the timing of VCE is one of the most important factors influencing its diagnostic yield.[5] The first study that suggested the importance of timing was that of Pennazio and colleagues,[10] who evaluated 100 consecutive patients with ongoing obscure-overt, previous obscure-overt, and ongoing OGIB. Diagnostic yield was highest in patients with ongoing obscure-overt bleeding (92.3%), then with ongoing obscure bleeding (44.2%), and last with prior bleeding (12.9%). Moreover, in patients with prior bleeding, the diagnostic yield was highest in patients with a shorter interval between last bleed and VCE. Although a 92% detection rate has never been reproduced, the data of Pennazio and colleagues[10] first suggested a larger role for VCE in acute bleeding more than a decade ago. Since then, additional studies have strengthened the role for expedited VCE. Immediate VCE within 48 hours of presentation can detect bleeding lesions in up to 73% to 87% of cases.[29] The rate of detection decreases progressively with increasing intervals of time from presentation, reaching as low as 35% if the capsule is deployed distant from the time of bleeding.[30] In one trial, VCE performed within 72 hours of presentation identified either active bleeding or an angioectasia in an additional 16% of patients than when performed after 72 hours. In addition, earlier VCE led to significantly more therapeutic interventions (18.9% vs 7.4%) and shorter lengths of admission (6.1 days vs 10.3 days).[31] Efforts should be made to perform VCE as early as possible, owing to higher rates of diagnosis and higher rates of surgical and endoscopic intervention achieved with earlier timing (**Figs. 1** and **2**).

Earlier timing of VCE also offers unique advantages as a risk stratification tool. Risk stratification is recommended among the major professional societies in order to triage cases of acute gastrointestinal bleeding and affect the timing of endoscopy. Traditional tools for risk stratification have included nasogastric tube (NGT) aspiration and clinical scoring calculators, such as the Blatchford and Rockall score.[1-3] NGT aspiration, which relies on the aspiration of stomach contents through the NGT, has since fallen out of favor because of poor predictive value and significant patient discomfort associated with placing the NGT. Likewise, poor test characteristics have limited the widespread clinical adoption of the Blatchford and Rockall scores. Compared with NGT aspiration, VCE detects blood more often (83.3% vs 33.3%) and might better facilitate patient triage to endoscopy.[32] Compared with the Blatchford and Rockall scoring calculators, VCE is more accurate in acute upper gastrointestinal bleeding (UGIB).[33] The negative predictive value of VCE for rebleeding is excellent, reaching up to 94%, which can provide reassurance and help to facilitate an earlier discharge following a negative evaluation.[18]

Earlier timing of VCE also offers cost advantages. Meltzer and colleagues[34] developed decision analysis software to compare the cost-effectiveness of various

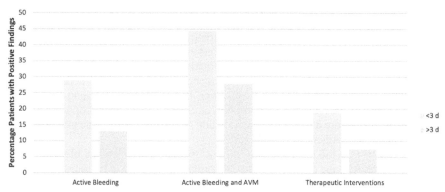

Fig. 1. Diagnostic yield and therapeutic yield of VCE in an inpatient cohort stratified by time of deployment. (*Data from* Singh et al. Timing of video capsule and endoscopy relative to overt obscure GI bleeding: implications from a retrospective study. Gastrointest Endosc. 2013;77(5):761 to 766.)

approaches to acute gastrointestinal bleeding. The software compared the overall cost and incremental quality-adjusted life years (QALYs) between direct imaging with VCE in the ED, risk stratification using the Blatchford score, risk stratification using NGT aspiration, and an all-admit approach. In low-risk patients, VCE was the preferred approach in terms of both cost and QALYs. In moderate-risk patients, use of VCE remained preferable to NGT aspiration, and was also more effective than the all-admit approach.[34]

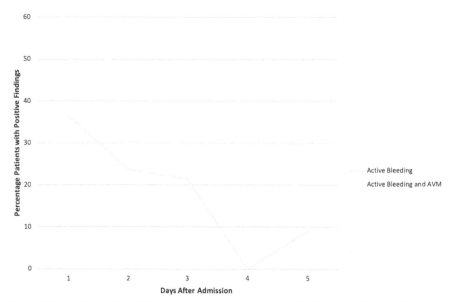

Fig. 2. Diagnostic yield of VCE in an inpatient cohort stratified by time since deployment. (*Data from* Singh et al. Timing of video capsule and endoscopy relative to overt obscure GI bleeding: implications from a retrospective study. Gastrointest Endosc. 2013;77(5):761 to 766.)

VIDEO CAPSULE ENDOSCOPY IN ACUTE GASTROINTESTINAL BLEEDING

The evaluation of acute gastrointestinal bleeding, which includes hematemesis and nonhematemesis gastrointestinal bleeding, has historically been within the domain of conventional endoscopy. Indeed, current guidelines do not routinely recommend VCE until after upper endoscopy and colonoscopy have excluded sources within reach of the conventional endoscope. However, this paradigm is starting to change. VCE, for example, has leapfrogged repeat or second-look endoscopy within the ESGE guidelines, where it holds a strong position as the third diagnostic test of choice in unidentified gastrointestinal bleeding.[28]

The role of VCE in the management of nonobscure gastrointestinal bleeding continues to evolve. Its ease of use, minimal risk profile, and ability to be rapidly administered in the acute care setting makes it an attractive option in the evaluation of all forms of gastrointestinal bleeding. Recent studies evaluating the use of VCE in the ED have demonstrated that the immediate use of VCE improves diagnostic and therapeutic outcomes and shortens length of admission. VCE might also be useful in the diagnosis of causes of noncardiac chest pain. VCE is more than capable of detecting bleeding lesions in the esophagus, stomach, and proximal small bowel with favorable testing characteristics. It has been demonstrated to be able to detect both angioectasias and gastric antral vascular ectasia within reach of a conventional endoscope, directing therapeutic interventions that resulted in favorable long-term outcomes in up to 80% of cases.[35,36]

VCE also compares favorably with conventional upper endoscopy in the detection of non–small bowel sources of bleeding. In one trial, VCE had equivalent rates of detection compared with upper endoscopy for peptic and inflammatory lesions (67.5% vs 87.5%).[32] In another small trial, all patients with suspected UGIB and positive findings for coffee grounds or blood on VCE had their findings confirmed on upper endoscopy, whereas in all 4 patients with negative findings on VCE, none had evidence of high-risk stigmata on subsequent endoscopy.[33]

Clinical trials have also validated the role of VCE in non–small bowel acute gastrointestinal bleeding, and there is now strong evidence from several randomized controlled trials (RCTs) that the use of VCE in the ED in these patients can improve clinical and patient-centered outcomes. In one RCT from Sung and colleagues,[37] 71 patients in the ED with suspected UGIB were randomized into either standard treatment at the discretion of the admitting doctor, or immediate VCE with admission determined by capsule findings. In the group that underwent VCE, just 7 patients were admitted compared with all 34 patients in the non-VCE group. Despite the lower rate of admission, there was no difference between each group in recurrent bleeding or 30-day mortality.[37] In a second RCT, this from Marya and colleagues,[38] 87 patients with suspected UGIB in the ED were randomized to either immediate VCE or standard of care. The main outcome was detection of active bleeding or stigmata of recent hemorrhage, which occurred in 64.3% of patients in the VCE arm compared with 31.1% of patients in the standard of care arm.[38] On close review of this trial, most of this benefit came from the improved identification of vascular lesions (19.0% in the VCE arm vs 4.4% in standard arm) and colonic bleeding (31.0% in the VCE arm vs 8.8% in the standard arm). This raises 2 important points. First, it highlights the importance of earlier timing. Vascular lesions are often small and difficult to diagnose. Angioectasias, for example, bleed intermittently and lack the characteristic high-risk stigmata of ulcers. Thus, it is difficult if not impossible for endoscopists to tell in the moment whether an angioectasia is the source of bleeding and has now stopped, or is a nonculprit coexistent lesion. Catching vascular lesions in the act of bleeding can thus lead to targeted interventions and reduce recurrent bleeding. Second, it highlights the capabilities of VCE as a tool to target therapeutic procedures. Highlighted here, in patients presenting with melena, significantly more patients in the capsule arm were found to have bleeding localized in the midgut or colon than in the standard of care arm. The conventional algorithm would put these patients through an esophagogastroduodenoscopy, followed with a colon-cleansing preparation, and then colonoscopy, perhaps occurring 48 to 72 hours after presentation. This would not just result in unneeded procedures, but in the time it takes to navigate the conventional algorithm to arrange a colonoscopy, the bleeding could have stopped or otherwise be washed away with the cleansing preparation, removing a clue as to the ultimate diagnosis. Further studies are of course warranted, given the strong evidence to date that VCE in the acute setting improves bleeding localization, leads to more rapid diagnoses, avoids unneeded procedures, and reduces admission rates without a detriment to overall survival or readmission rates.

VIDEO CAPSULE ENDOSCOPY IN SPECIAL CIRCUMSTANCES

Two circumstances deserve special mention with regard to the role of VCE. The first is in the evaluation of noncardiac chest pain in patients presenting to the ED. In the more than 6 million annual visits to the ED for chest pain, the acute coronary syndrome accounts for approximately 10% of visits. In the remaining patients, 20% to 60% will have esophageal mucosal disease diagnosed on upper endoscopy. In a prospective trial by Singh and colleagues,[39] use of PillCam ESO led to a diagnosis of esophageal disease in 38% of patients with noncardiac chest pain. The test was well tolerated, and no PillCam-related complications occurred. Although further research is needed, VCE has potential in the management of nonbleeding gastrointestinal conditions, such as esophagitis, and could lead to more rapid diagnoses, expedited discharge, reduced readmission rates, and better overall care.[39]

The second circumstance in which VCE holds promise as a diagnostic modality is in resource-constrained settings. Successful conventional endoscopy requires multiple participating parts, including the endoscopist, nurse, endoscopy tech, anesthesia team, and preoperative and postoperative care teams. In addition, resources must be spent on transporting the patient and recovering the patient, as well as on the required instruments and personal protective equipment (PPE). Perhaps never has this burden of resources been better highlighted than during the severe acute respiratory syndrome coronavirus 2 (SARS-CoV-2) pandemic, during which time hospitals around the globe struggled with maintaining the needed levels of PPE to protect their patients and their staff. Elective procedures were curtailed, and the timing of urgent procedures came under scrutiny, as one infected individual could place multiple individuals at risk, in particular during aerosol-generating procedures, such as endoscopy. In response to this problem, Hakimian and colleagues[40] have proposed an alternative approach to the current standard of care. In their approach, Hakimian and colleagues[40] prioritized VCE as a first-line diagnostic modality in gastrointestinal bleeding to reduce the number of interventions and limit resource utilization during the SARS-CoV-2 pandemic. Compared with the standard of care, patients who underwent first-line VCE experienced no differences in terms of overall mortality, rates of rebleeding, or readmissions for rebleeding. Moreover, patients who underwent first-line VCE required significantly fewer invasive procedures than in the standard of care (44% vs 96%). Bleeding localization was reached more often in the VCE-first arm (78% vs 72%), as was identification of active bleeding or stigmata or recent bleeding (66% vs 28%).[40] Similar results might be able to be extrapolated to other resource-limited settings, including weekends and holidays during which time staff is less available.

CLINICS CARE POINTS

- Early deployment of VCE in patients with gastrointestinal bleeding is critical in improving diagnostic yield.
- Data are accumulating for the use of VCE as a first-line diagnostic modality in the evaluation of both hematemesis and nonhematemesis gastrointestinal bleeding.
- VCE might be particularly useful in the evaluation and triage of patients with gastrointestinal bleeding in resource-limited settings, such as during a pandemic or during weekends.
- PillCam ESO in the evaluation of patients with noncardiac chest pain in the ED is both well tolerated and effective in the detection of esophagitis.

DISCLOSURE

There are no financial or commercial conflicts of interest to disclose among any of the authors.

REFERENCES

1. Hwang JH, Fisher DA, Ben-Menachem T, et al. The role of endoscopy in the management of acute non-variceal upper GI bleeding. Gastrointest Endosc 2012; 75(6):1132–8.
2. Laine L, Jensen DM. Management of patients with ulcer bleeding. Am J Gastroenterol 2012;107(3):345–60 [quiz 361].
3. Gralnek IM, Dumonceau J-M, Kuipers EJ, et al. Diagnosis and management of nonvariceal upper gastrointestinal hemorrhage: European Society of Gastrointestinal Endoscopy (ESGE) Guideline. Endoscopy 2015;47(10):a1–46.
4. Strate LL, Gralnek IM. ACG clinical guideline: management of patients with acute lower gastrointestinal bleeding. Am J Gastroenterol 2016;111(5):755.
5. Gerson LB, Fidler JL, Cave DR, et al. ACG clinical guideline: diagnosis and management of small bowel bleeding. Am J Gastroenterol 2015;110(9):1265–87 [quiz 1288].
6. Lau WY, Fan ST, Wong SH, et al. Preoperative and intraoperative localisation of gastrointestinal bleeding of obscure origin. Gut 1987;28(7):869–77.
7. Mylonaki M, Fritscher-Ravens A, Swain P. Wireless capsule endoscopy: a comparison with push enteroscopy in patients with gastroscopy and colonoscopy negative gastrointestinal bleeding. Gut 2003;52(8):1122–6.
8. Rondonotti E, Villa F, Mulder CJJ, et al. Small bowel capsule endoscopy in 2007: indications, risks and limitations. World J Gastroenterol 2007;13(46):6140–9.
9. Delvaux M, Fassler I, Gay G. Clinical usefulness of the endoscopic video capsule as the initial intestinal investigation in patients with obscure digestive bleeding: validation of a diagnostic strategy based on the patient outcome after 12 months. Endoscopy 2004;36(12):1067–73.
10. Pennazio M, Santucci R, Rondonotti E, et al. Outcome of patients with obscure gastrointestinal bleeding after capsule endoscopy: report of 100 consecutive cases. Gastroenterology 2004;126(3):643–53.

11. Katsinelos P, Lazaraki G, Gkagkalis A, et al. The role of capsule endoscopy in the evaluation and treatment of obscure-overt gastrointestinal bleeding during daily clinical practice: a prospective multicenter study. Scand J Gastroenterol 2014; 49(7):862–70.

12. Carey EJ, Leighton JA, Heigh RI, et al. A single-center experience of 260 consecutive patients undergoing capsule endoscopy for obscure gastrointestinal bleeding. Am J Gastroenterol 2007;102(1):89–95.

13. Lepileur L, Dray X, Antonietti M, et al. Factors associated with diagnosis of obscure gastrointestinal bleeding by video capsule enteroscopy. Clin Gastroenterol Hepatol 2012;10(12):1376–80.

14. Bresci G, Parisi G, Bertoni M, et al. The role of video capsule endoscopy for evaluating obscure gastrointestinal bleeding: usefulness of early use. J Gastroenterol 2005;40(3):256–9.

15. Ben Soussan E, Antonietti M, Hervé S, et al. Diagnostic yield and therapeutic implications of capsule endoscopy in obscure gastrointestinal bleeding. Gastroenterol Clin Biol 2004;28(11):1068–73.

16. Kim J-B, Ye BD, Song Y, et al. Frequency of rebleeding events in obscure gastrointestinal bleeding with negative capsule endoscopy. J Gastroenterol Hepatol 2013;28(5):834–40.

17. Koh S-J, Im JP, Kim JW, et al. Long-term outcome in patients with obscure gastrointestinal bleeding after negative capsule endoscopy. World J Gastroenterol 2013;19(10):1632–8.

18. Lai LH, Wong GLH, Chow DKL, et al. Long-term follow-up of patients with obscure gastrointestinal bleeding after negative capsule endoscopy. Am J Gastroenterol 2006;101(6):1224–8.

19. Macdonald J, Porter V, McNamara D. Negative capsule endoscopy in patients with obscure GI bleeding predicts low rebleeding rates. Gastrointest Endosc 2008;68(6):1122–7.

20. Viazis N, Papaxoinis K, Vlachogiannakos J, et al. Is there a role for second-look capsule endoscopy in patients with obscure GI bleeding after a nondiagnostic first test? Gastrointest Endosc 2009;69(4):850–6.

21. Cheifetz AS, Kornbluth AA, Legnani P, et al. The risk of retention of the capsule endoscope in patients with known or suspected Crohn's disease. Am J Gastroenterol 2006;101(10):2218–22.

22. Li F, Gurudu SR, De Petris G, et al. Retention of the capsule endoscope: a single-center experience of 1000 capsule endoscopy procedures. Gastrointest Endosc 2008;68(1):174–80.

23. Repici A, Barbon V, De Angelis C, et al. Acute small-bowel perforation secondary to capsule endoscopy. Gastrointest Endosc 2008;67(1):180–3.

24. Leung WK, Ho SSM, Suen B-Y, et al. Capsule endoscopy or angiography in patients with acute overt obscure gastrointestinal bleeding: a prospective randomized study with long-term follow-up. Am J Gastroenterol 2012;107(9):1370–6.

25. Saperas E, Dot J, Videla S, et al. Capsule endoscopy versus computed tomographic or standard angiography for the diagnosis of obscure gastrointestinal bleeding. Am J Gastroenterol 2007;102(4):731–7.

26. Triester SL, Leighton JA, Leontiadis GI, et al. A meta-analysis of the yield of capsule endoscopy compared to other diagnostic modalities in patients with obscure gastrointestinal bleeding. Am J Gastroenterol 2005;100(11):2407–18.

27. Douard R, Wind P, Berger A, et al. Role of intraoperative enteroscopy in the management of obscure gastointestinal bleeding at the time of video-capsule endoscopy. Am J Surg 2009;198(1):6–11.

28. Pennazio M, Spada C, Eliakim R, et al. Small-bowel capsule endoscopy and device-assisted enteroscopy for diagnosis and treatment of small-bowel disorders: European society of gastrointestinal endoscopy (ESGE) clinical guideline. Endoscopy 2015;47(4):352–76.

29. Goenka MK, Majumder S, Kumar S, et al. Single center experience of capsule endoscopy in patients with obscure gastrointestinal bleeding. World J Gastroenterol 2011;17(6):774–8.

30. Yamada A, Watabe H, Kobayashi Y, et al. Timing of capsule endoscopy influences the diagnosis and outcome in obscure-overt gastrointestinal bleeding. Hepatogastroenterology 2012;59(115):676–9.

31. Singh A, Marshall C, Chaudhuri B, et al. Timing of video capsule endoscopy relative to overt obscure GI bleeding: implications from a retrospective study. Gastrointest Endosc 2013;77(5):761–6.

32. Gralnek IM, Ching JYL, Maza I, et al. Capsule endoscopy in acute upper gastrointestinal hemorrhage: a prospective cohort study. Endoscopy 2013;45(1):12–9.

33. Gutkin E, Shalomov A, Hussain SA, et al. Pillcam ESO(®) is more accurate than clinical scoring systems in risk stratifying emergency room patients with acute upper gastrointestinal bleeding. Therap Adv Gastroenterol 2013;6(3):193–8.

34. Meltzer AC, Ward MJ, Gralnek IM, et al. The cost-effectiveness analysis of video capsule endoscopy compared to other strategies to manage acute upper gastrointestinal hemorrhage in the ED. Am J Emerg Med 2014;32(8):823–32.

35. Kitiyakara T, Selby W. Non-small-bowel lesions detected by capsule endoscopy in patients with obscure GI bleeding. Gastrointest Endosc 2005;62(2):234–8.

36. Sidhu R, Sanders DS, McAlindon ME. Does capsule endoscopy recognise gastric antral vascular ectasia more frequently than conventional endoscopy? J Gastrointest Liver Dis 2006;15(4):375–7.

37. Sung JJY, Tang RSY, Ching JYL, et al. Use of capsule endoscopy in the emergency department as a triage of patients with GI bleeding. Gastrointest Endosc 2016;84(6):907–13.

38. Marya NB, Jawaid S, Foley A, et al. A randomized controlled trial comparing efficacy of early video capsule endoscopy with standard of care in the approach to nonhematemesis GI bleeding (with videos). Gastrointest Endosc 2019;89(1):33–43.e4.

39. Sing A, Lee C, Finkelberg D, et al. A pilot study of the use of pill-cam ESO for esophageal disease in patients presenting to the emergency department with non cardiac chest pain. Gastroenterology 2010;135(5).

40. Hakimian S, Hanscom C, Petersile M, et al. Video capsule endoscopy as first procedure for acute gastrointestinal bleeding: an approach to minimizing exposure to SARS-CoV-2 and conserving resources. The American Journal of Gastroenterology 2020;115:S295.

The Role of Provocative Testing and Localization of the Video Capsule Endoscope in the Management of Small Intestinal Bleeding

Daniel L. Raines, MD[a],*, Douglas G. Adler, MD[b]

KEYWORDS

- Small intestinal bleeding • Provocative angiography • Provocative endoscopy
- Video capsule endoscopy • Device-assisted enteroscopy

KEY POINTS

- Cases of small intestinal bleeding (SIB) are commonly encountered in clinical practice despite advancements in medical technology that allow consistent visualization of the entire gastrointestinal tract.
- The use of antithrombotic agents to provoke bleeding has been found to be revealing in cases of SIB when used in combination with angiography as well as endoscopy.
- The performance of endoscopic procedures, including video capsule endoscopy (VCE) and device-assisted enteroscopy (DAE) on active antiplatelet and/or anticoagulant therapy is considered low risk and may improve diagnostic yield.
- The use of VCE for gastrointestinal bleeding in the inpatient setting has been found to improve diagnostic yield and decrease hospital stay.
- Because DAE is required for therapeutic intervention in patients with small bowel bleeding, access to this technology is essential for effective management in many cases.

 Video content accompanies this article at http://www.giendo.theclinics.com/.

OBSCURE GASTROINTESTINAL BLEEDING
Definitions

Small intestinal bleeding (SIB) has been described as bleeding that is undefined in cause despite evaluation by standard upper endoscopy, colonoscopy, and small bowel follow-through (SBFT). The low diagnostic yield of SBFT combined with the advent of higher-yield small bowel studies has resulted in the removal of SBFT from

[a] 1542 Tulane Avenue, Suite 423, New Orleans, LA, USA; [b] University of Utah School of Medicine, 30 North 1900 East 4R118, Salt Lake City, UT 84132, USA
* Corresponding author. 200 West Esplanade, Suite 200, Kenner, LA 70112.
E-mail address: draine@lsuhsc.edu

Gastrointest Endoscopy Clin N Am 31 (2021) 317–330
https://doi.org/10.1016/j.giec.2021.01.001
1052-5157/21/© 2021 Elsevier Inc. All rights reserved.

algorithms for evaluation of gastrointestinal (GI) bleeding.[1,2] Video capsule endoscopy (VCE) is associated with a 38% to 83% diagnostic yield in patients with suspected small bowel bleeding and is therefore recommended as the next step in management after negative esophagogastroduodenoscopy (EGD)/colonoscopy.[3] Computed tomography enterography (CTE) may be indicated after negative VCE, or as an alternative if VCE is contraindicated, and has a reported diagnostic yield of 40% in bleeding of suspected small bowel origin.[4,5] Device-assisted enteroscopy (DAE) by double balloon, single balloon, or spiral technique is a useful study in patients with suspected small bowel bleeding but is not available in all centers. Rates of total enteroscopy differ by technique but the diagnostic yield for all techniques is similar, around 60% to 80%.[6]

The widespread adoption of these advanced technologies to evaluate for small bowel bleeding sources resulted in a revision of definitions pertaining to obscure bleeding in 2015. Examples of bleeding with negative evaluation by EGD and colonoscopy are now termed suspected SIB. This group accounts for 5% of bleeding presentations, most of which are small bowel in origin.[7] Sources of blood loss in these cases can be grouped into lesions within the reach of standard endoscopy that are missed, accounting for 25% of sources, and lesions in the small intestine, accounting for 75%. The term obscure GI bleeding is now typically reserved for cases in which a bleeding source cannot be identified despite current standard-of-care evaluation, including EGD, colonoscopy, VCE, and/or DAE and radiographic studies.[2]

Distribution of Bleeding Sources

Missed lesions should be considered as lesions that are difficult to detect (**Table 1**), which includes lesions that are identifiable on closer inspection as well as vascular abnormalities, such as Dieulafoy lesions, which are difficult or impossible to detect unless actively bleeding (**Fig. 1**A, B).[8] Bleeding sources that are commonly missed on upper endoscopy include Cameron erosions, associated with a large hiatal hernia; gastric antral vascular ectasia, which may appear as benign mucosal erythema; small or concealed angioectasias (**Figs. 2** and **3**); and peptic ulcers that are positioned in a location difficult to visualize. Missed lesions on colonoscopy include flat neoplasms as well as angioectasias in the right colon. Missed lesions in the small bowel vary according to patient age. In patients older than 50 years, angioectasias are the most common cause of small bowel bleeding in the Western population and are the most common missed small bowel lesion by VCE.[2,9] In adults younger than 50 years, tumors of the

Table 1 Culprit sources in suspected small bowel bleeding		
Missed Lesions on Upper Endoscopy	*Small Bowel Bleeding Sources*	
Cameron erosions	Vascular lesions	Ulcerative disorders
Peptic ulcer disease	• Angioectasias	• Crohn disease
GAVE	• Dieulafoy lesion	• NSAID enteropathy
Angioectasias	• Aortoenteric fistula	• Ischemic enteropathy
Dieulafoy lesion	Neoplasms	• Radiation enteropathy
Missed lesions on colonoscopy	• Carcinoid	• Meckel diverticulum
Flat neoplasms	• GIST	
Angioectasias	• Adenocarcinoma	
Dieulafoy lesion	• Lymphoma	

Abbreviations: GAVE, gastric antral vascular ectasia; GIST, GI stromal tumor; NSAID, nonsteroidal antiinflammatory drug.

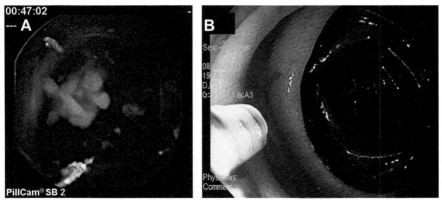

Fig. 1. (*A, B*) Small bowel Dieulafoy lesion observed by VCE then subsequent DAE.

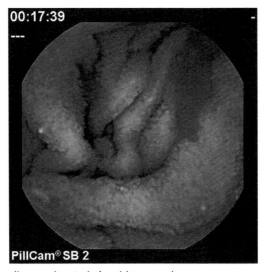

Fig. 2. Actively bleeding angioectasia by video capsule.

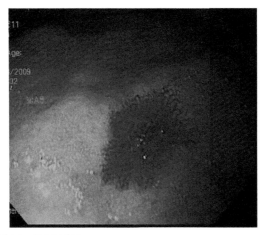

Fig. 3. Dense gastric angioectasias.

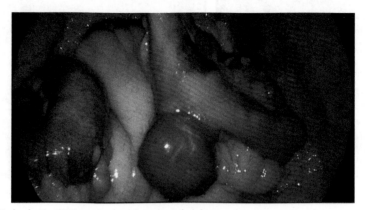

Fig. 4. Endophytic GIST marked with India ink (observed by laparoscopy).

small bowel are the most common bleeding source.[10] The miss rate of VCE for small bowel tumors is estimated to be 19%, especially for tumors such as GI stromal tumor (GIST) that can be endophytic (**Fig. 4**).[11] Therefore CTE is recommended after VCE in patients less than 50 years old or in patients more than 50 years old with recurrent bleeding or progressive anemia, although some tumors may remain undetected after both VCE and CTE (**Fig. 5**).[2,12] CTE may be combined with PET to show hypermetabolic lesions such as adenocarcinoma (**Fig. 6**A, B). A Meckel scan is recommended as an additional test, particularly in younger patients (**Fig. 7**).

Outcomes in Obscure Gastrointestinal Bleeding

Outcomes in patients with bleeding of unknown origin after negative EGD, colonoscopy, and VCE have been evaluated in several studies. Two early studies of SIB patient cohorts reported rebleeding rates of only 6% to 11% over an average 18-month follow-up period.[13,14] These studies also showed that negative capsule endoscopy (CE) was predictive of lower rebleeding rates compared with patients with positive CE. However, subsequent studies of this patient population conflict with these results. In 1 study, 26 patients with mostly overt obscure GI bleeding (OGIB) were followed over an extended median follow-up period of 32 months and rebleeding was observed in 35% of patients. In addition, this study found that rebleeding rates

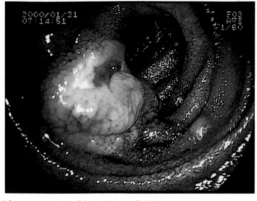

Fig. 5. Ileal carcinoid tumor missed by VCE and CTE.

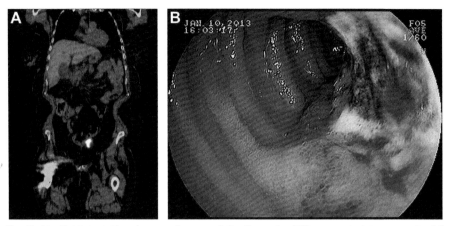

Fig. 6. (*A, B*) Metastatic adenocarcinoma of the ileum by PET–computed tomography (*A*) and DAE (*B*).

between patients with negative CE and positive CE were almost identical and only specific therapy directed to the bleeding source resulted in a change in the frequency of rebleeding.[15] Although this study was retrospective and complicated by a high rate of incomplete capsule examinations (67%), similar results were shown in another study of patients with SIB and negative CE.[16] This study found that 47% of patients with a nondiagnostic first CE study experienced recurrent overt bleeding or progressive anemia during a mean follow-up period of 25 months. Management of individual patients should therefore be tailored to the clinical course. In older patients with persistent resolution of bleeding, expectant management after negative VCE may be considered unless additional symptoms or clinical findings warrant further testing.[1,2] In younger patients and patients with recurrent overt bleeding or progressive anemia, additional testing should be pursued.

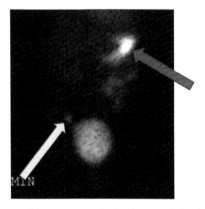

Fig. 7. Positive Meckel scan with tracer uptake in the gastric body (*red arrow*) and Meckel site (*yellow arrow*).

Repeat Testing in Obscure Gastrointestinal Bleeding

Additional testing in patients who experience progressive anemia attributed to GI blood loss or recurrent, overt bleeding after negative initial evaluation by EGD, colonoscopy, VCE, and/or DAE and CTE should be individualized. Supplemental history should be obtained, including previous history of epistaxis, blood donation, menstrual bleeding, frequent minor rectal bleeding, diarrhea, abdominal pain, history of radiation exposure, history of abdominal aortic aneurysm repair predisposing to aortoenteric fistula (**Figs.** 8 and **9**), nonsteroidal antiinflammatory drug use, olmesartan use, and family history of inflammatory bowel disease or celiac disease. After review of this additional history and previous studies, subsequent testing should be divided into 2 groups based on bleeding pattern as progressive anemia attributed to GI blood loss (occult bleeding) versus discrete episodes of hematochezia or melena (overt bleeding)

In patients with occult bleeding, repeat upper endoscopy with push enteroscopy is worthwhile to reevaluate for missed lesions in the upper GI tract as well as for angioectasias in the proximal small bowel and to obtain duodenal biopsies, if not previously performed.[17] Examination of the duodenum with a side-viewing duodenoscope may also be helpful in identifying bleeding sources in the duodenal wall or associated with the ampulla of Vater. Repeat colonoscopy with more extensive intubation of the terminal ileum can be considered to reevaluate for a flat neoplasm or angioectasias in the right colon as well as to further investigate for evidence of Crohn disease involving the distal ileum. In cases in which the initial CE study was incomplete or in which anemia is progressive, repeat CE should be considered. One study of second-look CE in 20 patients with occult bleeding reported a 35% diagnostic yield of a second CE.[18] Another study, which included 48 patients with occult, obscure bleeding, showed that repeat CE was successful in identifying a likely bleeding source in 65% of patients with progressive anemia, as defined by a 4-g/dL decrease in hemoglobin level. In patients who converted from occult to overt bleeding, the diagnostic yield of repeat CE was 100%.[16] If 1 or more of these studies is unrevealing, evaluation of the remaining small bowel through DAE should be pursued depending on availability. Intraoperative enteroscopy is the test of last resort in patients with severe anemia who have been evaluated by all other means.

Recurrent, overt SIB is often frustrating for both patients and clinicians but can usually be managed successfully with persistence. Repeated standard endoscopy, CE, angiography, and/or DAE should be performed as soon as possible after a

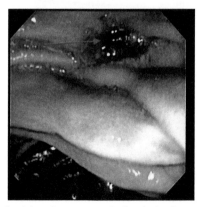

Fig. 8. Endoscopic view of a jejunal aortoenteric fistula (*red arrow*).

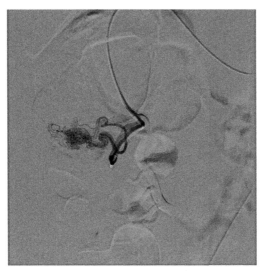

Fig. 9. Vascular tuft with early draining vein (*arrow*) consistent with AVM.

presentation with overt bleeding until bleeding stops or the bleeding site is localized. Multiple attempts may be required to successfully identify the bleeding source. Tagged red blood cell (RBC) scan is a useful adjunct to endoscopy because of its availability and lack of risk, although it is often unrevealing or nonspecific. Computed tomography angiography (CTA) may provide images that are easier to obtain and more localizing compared with tagged RBC scan. Patients with recurrent overt bleeding are considered to be the primary candidates for provocative testing.

PROVOCATIVE TESTING IN THE EVALUATION OF OBSCURE GASTROINTESTINAL BLEEDING

Provocation is defined as the introduction of a stimulus in attempt to elicit a specific response. Provocative testing is well established in the management of certain medical conditions, such as the stimulation of arrhythmias in electrophysiology.[19–21] Provocative angiography for the management of difficult cases of GI bleeding is included in the American Society for Gastrointestinal Endoscopy (ASGE) algorithm for evaluation of obscure GI bleeding but is practiced in a limited number of centers.[2] The use of provocation combined with endoscopy may be practiced in the community in low volumes but the current body of literature pertaining to this practice is limited to 4 case reports and 1 large retrospective study.[22–26] Although these techniques seem extreme, reported complication rates associated with these interventions are low, with reasonable diagnostic yields.[2]

Provocative Angiography

The body of literature pertaining to provocative angiography includes 9 series and 7 case reports totaling 126 cases (**Table 2**).[27–35] The first series published by Rosch and colleagues[27] in 1982 described 3 cases of recurrent, overt bleeding in which the administration of systemic heparin, intra-arterial heparin, and/or an intra-arterial vasodilator was used as an adjunct to conventional angiography with successful treatment of the bleeding source in all 3 cases. A subsequent study of provocation by Malden and colleagues[28] involved the administration of systemic heparin and systemic

Table 2
Provocative angiography case series

Series	Patients	Systemic Agents	Intra-arterial Agents	Success Rate (%)
Rosch et al,[27] 2017	3	Heparin	Tolazoline	100
Malden et al,[28] 1982	9	Heparin Urokinase	—	20
Koval et al,[29] 1998	10	Heparin	Tolazoline Streptokinase	80
Bloomfeld et al,[30] 1987	7	—	Heparin Tolazoline Urokinase	28
Ryan et al[31]	16	Heparin	Tolazoline tPA	37
Mernagh et al[32]	12	Heparin	—	50
Wildus et al[33]	9	—	Reteplase	89
Kim et al[34]	34	Heparin	Nitroglycerin tPA	31
Zurkiya et al[35]	19	—	Heparin Nitroglycerin tPA	26

Abbreviation: tPA, tissue plasminogen activator.

urokinase after initial negative mesenteric angiography followed by tagged RBC scan.[27] Positive tagged RBC scans were documented in 4 of 10 cases, but angiography was diagnostic in only 2 of these, resulting in an overall success rate of 20%. Systemic heparin alone was used in another study by Mernagh and colleagues[32] after initial negative angiography, which was associated with positive repeat angiography in 6 of 12 initial negative cases (yield of 50%). All of the remaining protocols have involved the use of systemic heparin accompanied by intra-arterial infusion of a vasodilator and/or thrombolytic, resulting in a wide range of diagnostic yields (18%–80%).[27–35] The 2 most recent case series of provocation using a combination of heparin, intra-arterial nitroglycerin, and intra-arterial tissue plasminogen activator (tPA) reported success rates of 26% to 31%.[34,35]

Despite concerns regarding the risk of bleeding associated with angiography in the setting of anticoagulation, the rate of complications in these reported series was low. Major complications were noted in only 3 of 126 cases. Rosch and colleagues[27] reported 1 episode of hematemesis during angiography after infusion of heparin, tolazoline, and streptokinase that stabilized with protamine infusion and transfusion of 2 units of blood. Koval and colleagues[29] reported 1 case of arterial wall puncture site hematoma after infusion of streptokinase. Kim and colleagues[34] reported 1 case of intestinal ischemia resulting in perforation requiring surgery after embolization of a lesion in the ileum, which was subsequently diagnosed as a carcinoid tumor during surgery.

The availability of mesenteric angiography varies by center according to the expertise and interest of the interventional radiology and interventional cardiology staff. The use of provocation combined with angiography is likely to be limited to interventionalists with a specific interest in and comfort level with mesenteric angiography. Mesenteric angiography is associated with risks of vascular injury, including hematoma and other bleeding complications, and these risks may be increased when combined with anticoagulant, antiplatelet, or thrombolytic agents. If an intervention such as embolization is planned, there is a risk of subsequent intestinal ischemia requiring surgery, which must be also be considered.

Provocative Endoscopy

The body of literature pertaining to provocative testing combined with endoscopy consisted of only 4 case reports before 2017. The first, by Berkelhammer and colleagues[22] in 2000, involved a 62-year-old man with an ileostomy who experienced recurrent overt bleeding. Upper endoscopy, ileoscopy, and provocative angiography were negative. Provocation with a 10,000-unit intravenous (IV) heparin bolus followed by a heparin 1000 unit/h infusion resulted in active bleeding 90 minutes later. Emergent ileoscopy subsequently revealed a Dieulafoy lesion 5 cm proximal to the stoma, which was treated definitively by distal ileal resection. In 2004, Wright and colleagues[23] described a 77-year-old man who presented with melena and hypotension resulting in intestinal ischemia and myocardial infarction. Repeat endoscopic testing and imaging by tagged RBC scan were negative for a bleeding source despite bleeding requiring transfusion of a total of 80 units of packed RBCs. Provocation with 5000 units of IV heparin resulted in active bleeding 2 hours later, indicated by bloody nasogastric tube output. Subsequent EGD revealed a Dieulafoy lesion in the stomach that was treated endoscopically. Reider and colleagues[24] published a case report in 2006 describing a 59-year-old man with a history of overt OGIB. EGD, colonoscopy, enteroclysis, push enteroscopy, and VCE did not identify a bleeding source. Provocative CE was performed with heparin IV infusion initiated 12 hours before the procedure and targeted to a partial thromboplastin time between 72 and 108 seconds (normal range, 26–36 seconds). Blood was observed in the proximal jejunum by VCE, and a subsequent laparotomy resulted in removal of a GIST. In addition, in 2007, Kumar and colleagues[25] published a case report of an unsuccessful provocative endoscopy attempt in a 65-year-old man presenting with hematochezia. Upper endoscopy and colonoscopy did not reveal a bleeding source. Tagged RBC scintigraphy localized the bleeding to the distal small bowel, whereas angiography localized the bleeding to the hepatic flexure; however, bleeding ceased and a lesion was not identified on subsequent colonoscopy despite provocation with 10,000 units of IV heparin and endoscopic observation for 75 minutes. The patient was taken to surgery, where a distal ileal carcinoid was found as the source of bleeding.

The authors published a retrospective review in 2017 of a databases of 824 DAE procedures. We identified 38 instances in which provocation with antiplatelet and/or anticoagulant agents was used as part of an OGIB evaluation in 27 patients.[26] Procedures were divided into 3 groups based on the method of provocation: cases in which an antiplatelet or anticoagulant agent was reintroduced because of a prior history of bleeding exacerbation related to this agent (provocation experienced); cases in which an antiplatelet or anticoagulant agent was administered without any such history (provocation naive); and extreme cases of recurrent, overt OGIB in which a combination of clopidogrel and IV heparin was administered for provocation (Louisiana State University (LSU) protocol). The diagnostic yield of provocative testing per procedure was 53% in the provocation-experienced group, 27% in the provocation-naive group, and 71% in the full-protocol group. Provocative testing was revealing in 15 out of 27 patients with angioectasias, and Dieulafoy lesions were found to be the most common lesions (Video 1). Provocative testing was not beneficial in 4 patients, who were eventually diagnosed with bleeding caused by intestinal angioectasias (3) and 1 patient with an aortoenteric fistula. The bleeding source was never found in 8 patients out of 27. There were no complications associated with any of the 38 procedures performed.

The ideal agent for provocative testing would have no adverse effects and would provoke bleeding consistently but not increase the risk of endoscopy. Antiplatelet agents such as clopidogrel are attractive because of evidence of platelet dysfunction being the culprit for precipitation of bleeding from angioectasias in several settings, such as bleeding from acquired von Willebrand factor deficiency in Heyde syndrome and in patients with left ventricular assist devices.[36,37] There is emerging evidence that endoscopy such as colonoscopy with polypectomy and DAE with argon plasma coagulation (APC) for treatment of angioectasias may be performed safely in the setting of active clopidogrel therapy.[38,39] If clopidogrel is selected as the stimulus, patients may be given a loading dose of 150 mg or 300 mg 8 hours before endoscopy in order to achieve 35% to 45% or 40% to 50% platelet inhibition, respectively.[40] In extreme cases of overt bleeding, a combination of clopidogrel and IV heparin may be considered to allow for both antiplatelet and anticoagulant effects with the ability to withdraw heparin (or reverse with protamine sulfate) resulting in endoscopy in the setting of clopidogrel alone. The use of systemic thrombolytic agents should be avoided because of the risk of major complication, such as stroke, associated with systemic administration of these agents and low yield observed in previous study of systemic thrombolytics.[28]

Many antiplatelet, anticoagulant, and antithrombotic agents have been introduced over the past 20 years. Each agent could be considered for inclusion in a provocation protocol depending on its effect, pharmacokinetics, and risk. One anticoagulant that might be considered for future protocols is dabigatran (Pradaxa), because a standard dose of 150 mg peaks in 2 hours and can be immediately reversed with IV infusion of idarucizumab (Praxbind).[41] Regarding antiplatelet agents, the glycoprotein IIb/IIIa inhibitor abciximab (ReoPro) can also be considered reversible because its short plasma half-life allows its hemostatic inhibition to be reversed with platelet administration.[42]

The ability of the endoscopist to reach the bleeding source is also a critical factor when considering provocative endoscopy, particularly when the bleeding segment has not been localized. The authors recommend that centers that might consider provocative endoscopy have the capability to perform total enteroscopy by DAE, preferably with double balloon enteroscopy. The ancillary resources of the center should also be assessed, including access to intensive care, angiography, and surgery services.

BLEEDING LOCALIZATION WITH VIDEO CAPSULE ENDOSCOPY

Accurate localization of the bleeding source is essential in CE interpretation. Experienced capsule readers can identify pitfalls in which the landmarks can be mislabeled, and small bowel transit times may be misleading. A fair estimate of the location of the bleeding segment can typically be made if the capsule transits through the entire small bowel. However, retention of the capsule endoscope in the duodenum for an extended period before transit through the deep small bowel is a source of confounding. The video capsule may reflux back and forth into the stomach after the first duodenal image. Residue or blood may interfere with proper delineation of landmarks as well as capsule transit. Early CE technology included a sensory array designed to show the capsule location in the abdomen in addition to obtaining images. However, this technology was abandoned with adoption of the sensor belt. CE technology has recently advanced to estimate progress more effectively through the small bowel by computer analysis of redundant images.[43] This software may still be fooled by inaccurate landmarks from the reader or by retention in the duodenum but shows promise for accurate assessment of location in most studies.

An experienced capsule reader may rely on the original study to determine an impression of where the lesion lies in the small bowel before intervening by DAE. A general rule for planning DAE after VCE is selection of an oral route for lesions observed in the first 60% of small bowel transit versus anal route for lesions observed in the last 40% of small bowel transit.[44,45] In some cases, DAE may be deferred if the abnormality observed on VCE appears to be within reach of standard upper endoscopy, push enteroscopy, or colonoscopy.

SUMMARY

Advances in techniques to evaluate bleeding sources have advanced to the point where obscure GI bleeding is now restricted to an estimated ~1% to 2% of all bleeding cases. However, in this small subset of patients, the bleeding source may remain undefined despite exhaustive testing. Where do clinicians go from here?

Attempts to intentionally stimulate bleeding for the purpose of identifying the bleeding source by angiography or endoscopy should be considered for select patients with recurrent, severe anemia or recurrent overt bleeding in whom exhaustive repeat testing is negative. A detailed discussion of the risks and benefits of provocative testing with the patients and their families is needed before attempting stimulation of bleeding. This discussion should include a review of the risks of angiography and/or endoscopy, which may be increased in the setting of active antiplatelet and/or anticoagulant therapy; the risk of stimulating bleeding that might not be successfully contained; and the increased risk of surgery in the event of uncontrollable bleeding or a procedure-related complication. However, provocative testing may be a justifiable intervention in highly selected cases in which the morbidity associated with recurrent bleeding justifies the additional risk.

VCE studies should be performed while maintaining routine antiplatelet and/or anticoagulant therapy. The performance of DAE as well as other endoscopic procedures should also be pursued on antithrombotics because these are considered low risk if diagnostic or include only APC and/or hemostatic clip placement.[46] Our study of DAE on active thienopyridine supports the safety and efficacy of this practice.[39] The performance of inpatient VCE may be limited in certain hospitals because of concerns about loss of capital. However, studies have shown that timely inpatient VCE significantly decreases hospital stay to offset the cost of the video capsule and improves diagnostic yield.[47]

In the future, advancements in artificial intelligence may allow computer localization of intestinal angioectasias, which may be present on only 1 of thousands of images.[48,49] These technologies may increase capture rate for this disorder and reduce read time. Progressive development of a motorized spiral enteroscope is an additional technology on the horizon that has been anxiously awaited by small bowel endoscopists because of its potential for rapid small bowel examination.[50]

DISCLOSURES

D.L. Raines: speaker and consultant for Medtronic. D.G. Adler: consultant/Advisory Board for BSC, Merit, Olympus; Speaker's Bureau for AbbVie.

SUPPLEMENTARY DATA

Supplementary video related to this article can be found at https://doi.org/10.1016/j.giec.2021.01.001.

REFERENCES

1. ASGE Standards of Practice Committee. The role of endoscopy in the management of obscure GI bleeding. Gastrointest Endosc 2010;72(3):471–9.
2. Gerson LB, Fidler JL, Cave DR, et al. ACG clinical guideline: diagnosis and management of small bowel bleeding. Am J Gastroenterol 2015;110(9):1265–87.
3. Rondonotti E, Villa F, Mulder CJ, et al. Small bowel capsule endoscopy in 2007: indications, risks and limitations. World J Gastroenterol 2007;13:6140–9.
4. Huprich JE, Fletcher JG, Fidler JL, et al. Prospective blinded comparison of wireless capsule endoscopy and multiphase CT enterography in obscure gastrointestinal bleeding. Radiology 2011;260(3):744–51.
5. Huprich JE, Fletcher JG, Alexander JA, et al. Obscure gastrointestinal bleeding: evaluation with 64-section multiphase CT enterography—initial experience. Radiology 2008;246(2):562–71.
6. Leighton JA. The role of endoscopic imaging of the small bowel in clinical practice. Am J Gastroenterol 2011;106:27–36.
7. Raju GS, Gerson L, Das A, et al. American gastroenterological association (AGA) Institute medical position statement on obscure gastrointestinal bleeding. Gastroenterology 2007;133:1694–6.
8. Tee HP, Kaffes AJ. Non-small-bowel lesions encountered during double-balloon enteroscopy performed for obscure gastrointestinal bleeding. World J Gastroenterol 2010;16(15):1885–9.
9. Regula J. Vascular lesions of the gastrointestinal tract. Best Pract Res Clin Gastroenterol 2008;22(2):313–28.
10. Lewis BS, Kornbluth A, Wayne JD. Small bowel tumors: yield of enteroscopy. Gut 1991;32:763–5.
11. Lewis BS, Eisen GM, Friedman S, et al. A pooled analysis to assess results of capsule endoscopy trials. Endoscopy 2005;37:960–5.
12. Boriskin HS, Devito BS, Hines JJ, et al. CT enterography vs capsule endoscopy. Abdom Imaging 2009;34:149–55.
13. Macdonald J, Porter V, McNamara D. Negative capsule endoscopy in patients with obscure GI bleeding predicts low rebleeding rates. Gastrointest Endosc 2008;68:1122–7.
14. Lai LH, Wong GL, Chow DK, et al. Long-term follow-up of patients with obscure gastrointestinal bleeding after negative capsule endoscopy. Am J Gastroenterol 2006;101:1224–8.
15. Park JJ, Cheon JH, Kim HM, et al. Negative capsule endoscopy without subsequent enteroscopy does not predict lower long-term rebleeding rates in patients with obscure GI bleeding. Gastrointest Endosc 2010;71(6):990–7.
16. Viazis N, Papaxoinis K, Vlachogiannakos J. Is there a role for second-look capsule endoscopy in patients with obscure GI bleeding after a nondiagnostic first test? Gastrointest Endosc 2009;69:850–6.
17. Lara LF, Bloomfield, Pineau BC. The rate of lesions found within reach of esophagogastroduodenoscopy during push enteroscopy depends on the type of obscure gastrointestinal bleeding. Endoscopy 2004;36:745–50.
18. Bar-Meir S, Eliakim R, Nadler M. Second capsule endoscopy for patients with severe iron deficiency anemia. Gastrointest Endosc 2004;60:711–3.
19. Spurrell RAJ, Krikler DM, Sowton E. Concealed bypasses of the atrioventricular node in patients with paroxysmal supraventricular tachycardia revealed by intracardiac stimulation and verapamil. Am J Cardiol 1974;33:590–5.

20. Denes P, Wu D, Dhingra RC, et al. Demonstration of dual AV nodal pathways in patients with supraventricular tachycardia. Circulation 1973;48:549–55.
21. Scheinman MM, Huang S. The NASPE prospective catheter ablation registry. Pacing Clin Electrophysiol 1998;23:1020–8.
22. Berkelhammer C, Radvany A, Lin A, et al. Heparin provocation for endoscopic localization of recurrent obscure GI hemorrhage. Gastrointest Endosc 2000;52: 555–6.
23. Wright CA, Petersen BT, Bridges CM, et al. Heparin provocation for identification and treatment of a gastric Dieulafoy's lesion. Gastrointest Endosc 2004;59: 728–30.
24. Rieder F, Schneidewind A, Bolder U, et al. Use of anticoagulation during wireless capsule endoscopy for the investigation of recurrent obscure gastrointestinal bleeding. Endoscopy 2006;38:526–8.
25. Kumar A, Gandolfo F, Halwan B. Provocation of bleeding during endoscopy in patients with recurrent acute lower gastrointestinal bleeding. Gastroenterol Hepatol 2007;3:570.
26. Raines DL, Jex K, Nicaud M, et al. Pharmacologic provocation combined with endoscopy in refractory cases of GI bleeding. Gastrointest Endosc 2017;85(1): 112–20.
27. Rosch J, Keller FS, et al. Pharmaco-angiography in the diagnosis of massive lower gastrointestinal bleeding. Radiology 1982;145:615–9.
28. Malden ES, Hicks ME, Royal HD, et al. Recurrent gastrointestinal bleeding: use of thrombolysis in diagnosis. Radiology 1998;207:147–51.
29. Koval G, Benner KG, Rösch J, et al. Aggressive angiographic diagnosis in acute lower gastrointestinal hemorrhage. Dig Dis Sci 1987;32:248–53.
30. Bloomfeld RS, Smith TP, Schneider AM, et al. Provocative angiography in patients with gastrointestinal hemorrhage of obscure origin. Am J Gastroenterol 2000; 95(10):2807–12.
31. Ryan JM, Key SM, Dumbleton SA, et al. Nonlocalized lower gastrointestinal bleeding. J Vasc Interv Radiol 2001;12:1273–7.
32. Mernagh JR, O'Donovan N, Somers S, et al. Use of heparin in the investigation of obscure gastrointestinal bleeding. Can Assoc Radiol J 2001;52(4):232–5.
33. Wildus DM. Reteplase provocative visceral angiography. J Clin Gastroenterol 2007;41:830–3.
34. Kim CY, Suhocki PV, Miller Jr MJ, et al. Provocative mesenteric angiography for lower gastrointestinal hemorrhage. J Vasc Interv Radiol 2010;21:477–83.
35. Zurkiya O, Ganguli S, Irani Z, et al. Provocative mesenteric angiography for gastrointestinal hemorrhage [abstract]. J Vasc Interv Radiol 25(3):S55.
36. Pate GE, Chandavimol M, Naiman SC, et al. Heyde's syndrome: a review. J Heart Valve Dis 2004;13:701–12.
37. Harvey L, Holley CT, John R. Gastrointestinal bleed after left ventricular assist device implantation: incidence, management, and prevention. Ann Cardiothorac Surg 2014;3:475–9.
38. Feagins LA, Uddin FS, Davila RE, et al. The rate of post-polypectomy bleeding for patients on uninterrupted clopidogrel therapy during elective colonoscopy is acceptably low. Dig Dis Sci 2011;56(9):2631–8.
39. Bollinger E, Spera M, Raines DL. The safety and efficacy of device-assisted enteroscopy in the setting of thienopyridine therapy. J Clin Gastroenterol 2017; 51(1):e1–e4.

40. Fukushima K, Yoshio K, Hideki K, et al. Effect of 150-mg vs 300-mg loading doses of clopidogrel on platelet function in japanese patients undergoing coronary stent placement. Circ J 2008;72:1282–4.

41. Pollack CV, Reilly PA, Eikelboom J, et al. Idarucizumab for dabigatran reversal. N Engl J Med 2015;373:511–20.

42. Tcheng JE. Clinical challenges of platelet glycoprotein IIb/IIIa receptor inhibitor therapy: bleeding, reversal, thrombocytopenia, and retreatment. Am Heart J 2000;139:S38–45.

43. Gomes S, Valerio MT, Salgo M, et al. Unsupervised neural network for homography estimation of capsule endoscopy frames. Procedia Computer Science 2019; 164:602–9.

44. Nakamura M, Ohimya N, Shirai O, et al. Route selection for double-balloon enteroscopy, based on capsule transit time, in obscure gastrointestinal bleeding. J Gastroenterol 2010;45(6):592–9.

45. Li X, Chen H, Dai J, et al. Predictive role of capsule endoscopy on the insertion route of double-balloon enteroscopy. Endoscopy 2009;41(9):762–6.

46. Acosta RD, Neena SA, Vinay C, et al. The management of antithrombotic agents for patients undergoing GI endoscopy. Gastrointest Endosc 2016;83(1):3–16.

47. Singh A, Marshall C, Chaudhuri B, et al. Timing of video capsule endoscopy relative to overt obscure GI bleeding: implications from a retrospective study. Gastrointest Endosc 2013;77:761–6.

48. Leenhardt R, Pauline V, Cynthia L, et al. A neural network algorithm for detection of GI angioectasia during small-bowel capsule endoscopy. Gastrointest Endosc 2018;89(1):189–94.

49. Alagappan M, Brown JRG, Mori Y, et al. Artificial intelligence in gastrointestinal endoscopy: the future is almost here. World J Gastrointest Endosc 2018;10: 239–49.

50. Mans L, Arvanitakis M, Neuhaus H, et al. Motorized spiral enteroscopy for occult bleeding. Dig Dis 2018;36:325–7.

Role of Video Capsule Endoscopy as a Prelude to Deep Enteroscopy

Dejan Micic, MD[a], Carol E. Semrad, MD[b],*

KEYWORDS

- Small bowel • Capsule endoscopy • Enteroscopy

KEY POINTS

- Video capsule endoscopy and device-assisted enteroscopy are complementary technologies.
- Capsule endoscopy is a highly acceptable technology with high diagnostic yield that can guide a subsequent enteroscopy approach.
- This article aimed to focus on the role of video capsule endoscopy as a prelude to deep enteroscopy with a focus on the strengths and limitations of either approach.

 Video content accompanies this article at http://www.giendo.theclinics.com.

INTRODUCTION

The small bowel is a challenge for endoscopic evaluation and therapy due to its length, angulated configuration, and limited tools when compared with the esophagus, stomach, and colon. Over the past 15 years, advances in endoscopy and radiologic imaging have provided the gastroenterologist new technologies to evaluate and treat small bowel disease, in particular the most commonly encountered problem of suspected small bowel bleeding. The development of video capsule endoscopy (VCE) has allowed for earlier diagnosis of small bowel bleeding with cost savings and excellent patient acceptance; however, it does not allow tissue sampling or therapy and the inability to control the capsule limits the examination. Device-assisted enteroscopy (DAE) has revolutionized small bowel bleeding therapy. It allows for treatment of vascular lesions and polyps and marking of tumors and ulcerating lesions for minimally

Competing Interests: Carol E. Semrad.
[a] Division of Internal Medicine, Section of Gastroenterology, Hepatology and Nutrition, University of Chicago, 5841 South Maryland Avenue, S401 MC 4076, Chicago, IL 60637, USA;
[b] Division of Internal Medicine, Section of Gastroenterology, Hepatology and Nutrition, University of Chicago, 5841 South Maryland Avenue, S401 MC 4080, Chicago, IL 60637, USA
* Corresponding author.
E-mail address: csemrad@medicine.bsd.uchicago.edu

Gastrointest Endoscopy Clin N Am 31 (2021) 331–344
https://doi.org/10.1016/j.giec.2020.12.008

invasive surgical resection. Due to the time and resource intensive nature of DAE, preceding VCE allows for a minimally invasive approach and is complementary to DAE in the diagnosis of small bowel pathology. This review focuses on the role of VCE before DAE in the clinical management of small bowel diseases.

DEVICE-ASSISTED ENTEROSCOPY

The small bowel is a relatively new territory for endoscopic diagnosis and treatment of disease. Limited methods have been historically used to evaluate the small bowel. Sonde enteroscopy was time and labor intensive without the capacity for therapy. Push enteroscopy allows for diagnosis and therapy of lesions, but evaluation is limited to the proximal jejunum (on average 80 cm beyond the ligament of Treitz).[1]

Wireless capsule endoscopy was the first technology that allowed for examination of the entire small bowel intestinal surface with high diagnostic yield that was noninvasive and had high patient acceptance. However, an inability to perform therapy or tissue sampling or control the passage of the capsule remain limitations.

Double balloon enteroscopy (DBE) was the first device developed that allowed for both diagnosis and therapy of lesions deep in the small bowel.[2] Using a 200-cm flexible enteroscope back-loaded on a 145-cm overtube with latex balloons on both ends, the small bowel in the abdominal cavity beyond the ligament of Treitz can be examined and then pleated onto the overtube in repetitive push-and-pull cycles.[3] In a prospective study of suspected small bowel bleeding, DBE demonstrated a greater insertion depth (230 + 100 cm vs 80 + 18 cm, $P<.0001$) and greater diagnostic yield (73% vs 44%) when compared with push enteroscopy.[1]

Other device-assisted technologies have since been developed with the goal of decreasing set-up time, lessening the need for specialized equipment, or reducing procedure time. Single balloon enteroscopy (SBE) uses a single balloon on the end of the overtube, allowing for decreased set-up time. In a randomized prospective trial comparing SBE and DBE, rates of complete enteroscopy were higher for DBE when compared with SBE (66% vs 22%, $P<.0001$), in general due to less slippage of the pleated bowel off of the overtube when deep in the small intestine with the DBE system; however, diagnostic yields were similar (52% vs 42%, $P = .42$).[4]

Spiral enteroscopy (SE) is a novel device that uses rotational energy to pleat bowel onto an overtube with spiral ridges at the tip that is attached to a pediatric colonoscope.[5] With clockwise rotation of the overtube, the small bowel past the ligament of Treitz is rapidly pleated. In a US study, SE was performed with a mean procedure time of 41 + 15 minutes and a diagnostic yield of 59%[6]; faster than procedure times for both DBE or SBE. When compared with SBE, the diagnostic yield of SE was not significantly different (59.6% vs 43.4%, $P = .12$).[7]

The newest device is a through-the-scope balloon system that uses a balloon catheter through the channel of a standard endoscope to advance into the small bowel. In one small study, both the antegrade and retrograde approaches into the small bowel were estimated to advance deeper than standard push enteroscopy and ileoscopy. Diagnostic yield was 44% and average advancement time was 15.5 minutes.[8] When comparing the technologies, DBE has the advantage of the deepest and most secure advancement in the small bowel, SBE has the fastest set-up time, and SE is the quickest to perform.

Small bowel radiologic imaging techniques have improved in parallel to include computed tomography (CT) and magnetic resonance (MR) enterography with mesenteric angiography, allowing for a unique evaluation of the small bowel wall for mass lesions, thickening, and vascular lesions.

Given the advances in endoscopic and cross-sectional evaluations of the small intestine, intraoperative enteroscopy is now reserved for those with incomplete evaluation of the small bowel and a high suspicion for a small bowel lesion. It can be performed minimally invasively using laparoscopic surgical assistance combined with DAE.[9]

APPROACH TO SMALL BOWEL DISEASES

The most common indication for evaluation of the small bowel is suspected bleeding. Approximately 5% of patients presenting with gastrointestinal bleeding (GIB) have no definite source found on upper endoscopy and colonoscopy,[10–12] and therefore have suspected small bowel bleeding. In approximately 75% of these patients, lesions can be identified in the small bowel using new endoscopic technologies.[11] Flat vascular lesions are the most common cause of small bowel bleeding in Western societies. Angioectasias (angiodysplasias) occur in association with disorders such as severe heart disease, chronic kidney disease, rheumatologic disorders, and cirrhosis,[13,14] and most commonly present as occult bleeding or iron deficiency anemia in individuals older than 60 years.

Other bleeding lesions in the small bowel include ulcers (most commonly due to nonsteroidal anti-inflammatory drug [NSAID] use, Crohn disease, radiation, ischemia, tuberculosis infection, nonspecific chronic ulcer, refractory celiac disease), tumors (gastrointestinal stromal tumor, neuroendocrine, lymphoma, adenocarcinoma), polyps (hamartoma, granulation, inflammatory, adenomas), hemangiomas, and diverticula (small bowel and Meckel). Synthesis of the clinical presentation, risk factors, and findings on prior endoscopic and cross-sectional imaging is critical for diagnosis, as both missed lesions and misinterpreted lesions can lead to clinical harm or overtreatment, respectively.

The suspected etiology of small bowel bleeding guides diagnostic testing and management. Most small bowel bleeding is undramatic in presentation and presents as stable or intermittent overt bleeding or occult bleeding with iron deficiency anemia (IDA). Although VCE is often the best test for the evaluation of small bowel bleeding in the setting of an overt bleeding presentation following a negative evaluation with upper and lower endoscopy, its use should be guided by a risk factor assessment.[15] Clinical history that includes type of bleeding, age, underlying medical conditions, medications, and presence of obstructive-type symptoms, physical examination, and laboratory testing can help elucidate the potential etiologies of small bowel pathology for cost-effective testing and to improve clinical outcomes. Chronic kidney disease, congestive heart failure, aortic stenosis, smoking, and pulmonary disease increase the risk of bleeding from small bowel angioectasias best detected by VCE. A personal history of melanoma, breast cancer, or kidney cancer increases the possibility of distant metastatic disease to the small bowel that may be missed on VCE and may be best evaluated on cross-sectional imaging in younger patients. A prior history of intra-abdominal surgery allows for identification of altered intestinal anatomy as well as risk of adhesions or stricture formation, which needs to be considered before undergoing VCE. Medication use should focus on the use of NSAIDs with respect to ulcer and stricture formation risk and antiplatelet and anticoagulant therapies that can accelerate the rate of small bowel bleeding. Physical examination can also guide clinical presentation, as hyperpigmented macules on the lips suggest Peutz-Jeghers syndrome and telangiectasis on the tongue suggests a diagnosis of hereditary hemorrhagic telangiectasia.

In suspected small bowel bleeding with an occult presentation, laboratory testing should focus on the diagnosis of IDA.[16] Although fecal occult blood testing (FOBT) has poor sensitivity for predicting causes of IDA[17] and is currently not recommended in the standard evaluation of IDA,[18] more recent studies suggest a role for FOBT in the setting of occult GIB with respect to suspected small bowel pathology,[19,20] although additional work is required to improve the sensitivity of FOBT for small bowel bleeding.[21]

VIDEO CAPSULE ENDOSCOPY AND DEVICE-ASSISTED ENTEROSCOPY: COMPLEMENTARY TECHNOLOGIES

VCE has a significantly higher diagnostic yield when compared with push enteroscopy (72.5% vs 48.7%, $P<.05$) in obscure GIB, particularly in the distal small bowel and for the detection of vascular lesions (62.5% vs 36.8%, $P = .05$).[22] In a prospective study comparing VCE with DBE, VCE detected more small bowel abnormalities (80% vs 60%, $P = .01$) and was more acceptable to the patient. However, DBE allowed for biopsy or intervention in 77% of performed studies.[23] A meta-analysis of 11 studies compared the overall yield of VCE with DBE and showed similar diagnostic yields (60% and 57%, respectively).[24] In a study comparing the diagnostic yield of VCE and DBE in 74 patients, the overall yield was not significantly different (VCE: 54% vs DBE: 64%); however, the discordant patient results demonstrated the limitations of either approach. Among individuals with a positive VCE and negative DBE (n = 4), all 4 patients had inaccessible bowel at DBE due to adhesions or peritoneal disease. Similarly, among individuals with a positive DBE and negative VCE (n = 11), bleeding was secondary to failure of detection of proximal small bowel lesions, Roux-en-Y anatomy and diverticula (Meckel and proximal small bowel diverticula).[25]

VIDEO CAPSULE ENDOSCOPY AS A PRELUDE TO DEVICE-ASSISTED ENTEROSCOPY IN GASTROINTESTINAL BLEEDING

DAE is invasive, time-consuming, and requires considerable resources. Given comparable yields, less invasiveness, and better patient acceptance, VCE has been recommended as the initial diagnostic test in suspected small bowel bleeding.[24] Performance of VCE before DAE facilitates detection of small bowel lesions, allows planning for the DAE approach, and increases the diagnostic yield of DAE[26] (Video 1).

In a cost-effectiveness model for the diagnosis and management of obscure GIB, 5 competing modalities (push enteroscopy, intraoperative enteroscopy, angiography, anterograde DBE, and VCE followed by DBE) were compared with a reference arm of no treatment with respect to total costs and quality-adjusted life years over a 1-year time period. An initial anterograde DBE was the most cost-effective and resulted in a higher bleeding cessation rate when compared with VCE (86% vs 76%). However, when considering the higher complication rate for DBE, VCE guiding DBE performance was the preferred approach.[27]

In a post hoc analysis of total direct costs of a randomized controlled trial comparing early VCE with a standard of care approach in nonhematemesis GIB,[28] no differences in direct costs or hospital length of stay were identified. However, VCE as the first diagnostic study demonstrated a greater diagnostic yield (69.2% vs 27.9%) that allowed a more directed approach to subsequent endoscopy. It was projected that early use of VCE in the emergency department with expedited discharge of individuals with negative studies has the potential to reduce costs and inpatient resource utilization.[28]

In a cost-effectiveness modeling study, placement of VCE for GIB in the emergency department was compared with clinical risk stratification and nasogastric tube placement as a diagnostic strategy and an admit-all strategy. In both mild and moderate upper GIB risk, VCE was the preferred strategy with respect to cost-effectiveness,[29] primarily directed by the high sensitivity of VCE in upper GIB,[30] allowing for discharge home without incurring the costs of hospital admission.

OPTIMIZING YIELD OF VIDEO CAPSULE ENDOSCOPY BEFORE DEVICE-ASSISTED ENTEROSCOPY

VCE has a high diagnostic yield for small bowel bleeding lesions but the accuracy of capsule reading depends on various factors (competence, clinical factors, completeness of study). It is equally important to know lesions that have been reported to be missed by capsule endoscopy. There are no landmarks deep in the small bowel to determine lesion location on VCE, thus lesion location relative to capsule transit time in the small bowel is useful in planning the DAE approach. A high positive predictive value >90% was reported when the lower DBE approach was reserved for capsule lesions found greater than 75% of the transit time from swallow to cecum[31] or greater than 60% of small bowel transit time from pylorus to ileocecal valve.[32] Similarly, in one small study, lesions identified within 50% to 60% of small bowel transit time from the duodenal bulb to the cecum were successfully reached in 100% of cases via the upper approach.[33] Lesion localization is much more difficult when the capsule has not reached the cecum by the end of the study. In such cases, fold pattern or increased vascularity of mucosa in the ileum may be helpful guides.

Role of Second-Look Endoscopy

Small bowel bleeding is often suspected following a negative evaluation on careful upper endoscopy and colonoscopy. Although a "second-look" endoscopy has been previously recommended based on literature documenting a miss rate of 2% to 25% on upper endoscopy and 6% to 23% on colonoscopy,[34] more recent clinical guidelines recommend VCE as the next diagnostic step in overt GIB.[15] As time to VCE is critical in improving diagnostic yield, and bleeding lesions outside of the small bowel can be evaluated on VCE, performance of repeat endoscopy in all referred cases of small bowel bleeding has not been found to be cost-effective.[35]

Factors that Impact Video Capsule Endoscopy Yield

Clinical factors

Factors predictive of a positive VCE study include overt bleeding, male sex, age older than 60, and inpatient capsule performance within 3 days of admission.[36–38] Those with ongoing overt bleeding have a higher diagnostic yield (92.3%) when compared with individuals with prior overt bleeding (12.9%) or those with positive FOBT or IDA (44.2%).[39] Age and male sex have been associated with the development of angioectasias,[37,40–42] whereas small bowel diverticular disease and Crohn disease are more common in those younger than 40 years.[43] Antiplatelet and anticoagulant use has been associated with small bowel bleeding[44] and continuation of therapy before VCE leads to an increase in positive findings,[45,46] thereby increasing the diagnostic yield of the study when performed to assess for bleeding lesions. When performed in an inpatient center, early use of VCE (<3 days from admission) is associated with an increased finding of angioectasia or bleeding, an increased rate of therapeutic intervention, and a shorter length of hospital stay.[38]

Timing of examination

Time to VCE is one of the most important factors in the diagnosis of small bowel bleeding lesions and timely therapeutic interventions. Two recent studies evaluated the role of early VCE in clinical bleeding presentations. In one small study of overt GIB (melena or maroon stools) and negative upper endoscopy, 20 patients underwent emergency VCE (within 24 hours of presentation). VCE correctly guided the diagnosis and subsequent therapeutic procedures in 17 patients (85%).[47] Fifteen patients (75%) had blood or a bleeding source identified within the small bowel (n = 11) or colon (n = 4). Prior studies of emergency VCE included only individuals undergoing both upper and lower endoscopy[48] and demonstrated the guidance of further diagnostic and therapeutic procedures in 78% of patients. Additional work is required to determine the impact on resource utilization of emergency VCE in active bleeding presentations.

In a recent randomized controlled trial, early VCE in GIB without hematemesis significantly improved diagnostic yield.[49] Early VCE (median 6 hours after presentation) compared with standard of care (upper endoscopy, capsule endoscopy, and/or colonoscopy) was more likely to localize a bleeding source (64.3% vs 31.1%, $P<.01$), identify a colonic source of bleeding (odds ratio [OR] 4.09, 95% confidence interval [CI] 1.12–15), have a presumptive diagnosis by the end of the admission (OR 2.67, 95% CI 0.95–7.47) and identify a vascular lesion as the source of bleeding (OR 10.73, 95% CI 1.6–72.11).[49] No differences were demonstrated in direct hospitalization costs or 30-day rebleeding risk. These novel studies are pushing the boundaries of VCE to detection of bleeding sources outside of the small bowel, which may impact the time to diagnosis and therapy. The impact on cost savings or rebleeding risk requires further study.

Reading competence
VCE is a unique technology that lacks the capacity for control, washing, insufflation, and sampling that facilitates interpretation of lesions by standard endoscopy. The capsule reader often is not the endoscopist performing DAE for therapy that limits the learning curve for capsule reading. Understanding capsule movement in the small intestine requires knowledge of the rapid motility in the duodenum that can lead to missed lesions and of the to-and-fro peristalsis that causes capsule tumbling allowing for misinterpretation of lesions (pylorus or ampulla as a mass lesion) or the number of lesions present (vascular, ulcerating, or polypoid). Field of view and capsule tumbling is thought to contribute to missed isolated mass lesions or jejunal and Meckel diverticula. Magnification is also higher on capsule endoscopy than standard endoscopy with the risk of reading artifacts as lesions (red spots as vascular lesions, air bubble as polyp, lens pressing against mucosa, or mucous as an ulcer).[50] This results in unnecessary DAE. Performance of DAE after VCE review by the same gastroenterologist improves capsule reading, interpretation of artifacts, and recognition of the wide variety of pathologies that can present in the small bowel.

SMALL BOWEL TUMORS

Small bowel neoplasms are found on VCE of the small bowel in 2.4%[51] to 9.5%[52] of studies, most often presenting with suspected small bowel bleeding (Video 2). Although more than 40 different histologic types of tumors are diagnosed in the small intestine, only 3% to 6% of all gastrointestinal neoplasms develop in the small intestine.[53] The rapid epithelial turnover rate, abundant lymphoid tissue, rapid transit through the small intestine, neutral pH, and immunoglobulin secretion are all hypothesized reasons as to the low burden of gastrointestinal neoplasms in the small bowel.[53] Among malignant tumors, neuroendocrine tumors are the most prevalent, followed by adenocarcinoma, lymphoma, and sarcoma.[54] Although most tumors are diagnosed unexpectedly in an evaluation of GIB, patients may present with obstructive symptoms due to luminal narrowing or intussusception or weight loss in the setting of metastatic disease. Suspicious findings on radiologic imaging studies and PET is more commonplace in the setting of evaluations for metastatic disease. Specific high-risk groups include longstanding inflammation in the small intestine secondary to celiac disease or Crohn disease and specific inherited syndromes to include familial adenomatous polyposis and Peutz-Jeghers syndrome, for which specific screening recommendations exist.[55,56]

Small bowel mass lesions have previously been demonstrated to have a high miss rate on VCE when compared with DBE and CT scan. In a retrospective review including 183 DBE procedures for obscure GIB, 18 small bowel mass lesions were identified. Among patients with mass lesions, 15 had a prior VCE, among which the mass lesion was identified in 5 (33%) and in which blood was identified in 7 (44%) without an associated mass lesion.[57] Although vascular lesions are typically multiple and present throughout the small bowel, mass lesions are often single and therefore can be missed due to the speed of the tumbling of the capsule in the small bowel. In addition, collapsed bowel, air bubbles, and preparation quality can all contribute to the miss rate for mass lesions in the small bowel.

In a pooled analysis of early studies using VCE, Lewis and colleagues[58] identified a miss rate for small bowel pathology of 10%, ranging from 0.5% for ulcers, 5.9% for vascular lesions, and 18.9% for small bowel neoplasms. Using a national cancer registry, Zagorowicz and colleagues[59] identified 15 small bowel tumors among 150 examinations for overt and occult obscure GIB. Over a median follow-up of 3.2 years, 3 missed small bowel masses were identified (2 gastrointestinal stromal tumors, 1 mesenteric tumor), providing a sensitivity of VCE of 83.3% for tumor detection.

Given the miss rate for mass lesions in the small bowel, VCE and CT enterography (CTE) are complementary strategies for diagnosis. A prospective study including 52 patients presenting with potential small bowel bleeding underwent VCE and triple-phase CT enterography within a 1-week interval. The diagnostic yields of VCE and CTE were 59.6% and 30.8% ($P = .004$), whereas the sensitivities for lesion detection of either evaluation were 72.2% and 44.4% ($P = .052$), respectively.[60] Importantly, the combined sensitivity of VCE and CTE increased to 88.9%, which was significantly greater than VCE or CTE alone. Specific to mass lesions, CTE demonstrated a sensitivity of 100% as compared with 66.7% for VCE. In a logistic regression analysis, individuals with an age younger than 40 and those presenting with severe bleeding had a higher diagnostic yield for CTE.

RETENTION/STRICTURE

The primary complication of VCE is capsule retention, defined as presence of the capsule within the digestive tract for at least 2 weeks after ingestion that requires further intervention[61] (Video 3). In a single retrospective study of 5593 capsules, the retention rate was 0.3%.[62] Higher rates have been reported in those with suspected Crohn disease (1.6%) or known Crohn disease (13%).[63] Other factors associated with strictures and a retained capsule include diaphragm disease from NSAID use[64] and radiation therapy.[65] Small bowel barium studies are of virtually no value in the prediction of capsule retention, whereas CT and MR enterography improve the ability to detect small bowel wall thickening and identify those at risk for retention.[3] In small bowel Crohn disease, capsule retention is associated with stricture length and the number of prestenotic dilations.[66] A dissolvable patency capsule predicts capsule retention in Crohn disease with known strictures that has led to safe performance of VCE in patients with obstructive-type symptoms and prior passage of a patency capsule.[67]

Although capsule retention in the small bowel may warrant surgery, DAE is the primary method for retrieval,[68] with a pooled successful retrieval rate of 86.5% (95% CI 75.6%–95.1%).[69] In the setting of a retained VCE, endoscopic balloon dilation of benign strictures can result in successful VCE removal as well as reduction in the need for future surgery, albeit at the cost of risk of perforation.[69]

THERAPEUTIC LONG-TERM IMPACT OF DEVICE-ASSISTED ENTEROSCOPY

High rates of rebleeding, similar to that of intraoperative enteroscopy or surgical resection, have been reported following therapeutic DBE for small bowel vascular lesions. Rebleeding rates range from 23% to 46%[70–72] depending on the duration of follow-up. In a pooled analysis of patients undergoing DBE for obscure GIB with a mean follow-up time of 26 ± 15 months, the rebleeding rate was 45%.[14] Risk factors for rebleeding include cardiac disease, chronic renal failure, cirrhosis, anticoagulation, number of vascular lesions, and presentation with overt bleeding.[71,72] Although a prior randomized study comparing an evaluation of VCE with small bowel radiography in obscure GIB failed to demonstrate a difference in rebleeding rate over 12 months between the 2 diagnostic methods, only 4 of 20 individuals with a positive VCE underwent DBE to allow for subsequent therapy in the small bowel.[73] A subsequent multicenter real-world cohort study demonstrated a high risk of rebleeding in individuals with a positive VCE that did not undergo therapeutic intervention.[74] Multiple therapeutic procedures for vascular lesions with rebleeding may be required for improved long-term outcomes,[75] and discontinuation of anticoagulation following VCE has been associated with a decreased risk of rebleeding.[76]

Clinical risk factors have now been incorporated into various risk scores to predict rebleeding. Female gender, cirrhosis, coumadin use, overt bleeding, and positive VCE findings have a high accuracy (C-statistic 0.733) over a median follow-up of 18.3 months.[77] The more recently described RHEMITT score assessed rebleeding risk over 12 months and includes the predictors of: renal disease, heart failure, tobacco use, VCE findings, major bleeding, and endoscopic treatment with high accuracy (C-statistic 0.842) in the initial study[78] and on external validation (C-statistic 0.756).[79] Although predictive, these risk scores have not been evaluated in the management of individuals with small bowel bleeding with respect to medical therapies to reduce the subsequent risk of rebleeding events.

Role of Second-Look Video Capsule Endoscopy

Whereas individuals with a positive VCE have a high risk of rebleeding, a negative VCE study is associated with a low rate of rebleeding ranging from 5.6% to 16.7%[80,81] in follow-up ranging from 19 months to 3 years. In a meta-analysis including 26 studies and 3657 individuals undergoing VCE, the pooled rate of rebleeding among those with a negative VCE was 19% (95% CI 14–25), which was significantly lower when compared with individuals with a positive VCE (29%, 95% CI 23–36; OR 0.59, 95% CI 0.37–0.95).[82]

Although bleeding lesions in the small bowel have a low miss rate on VCE,[58] and individuals with a negative VCE for obscure gastrointestinal bleeding (OGIB) have a low rate of rebleeding,[83] small bowel vascular lesions have the potential to intermittently bleed. In the event of recurrent overt bleeding, significant drop in hemoglobin, or poor visualization on initial capsule study, repeat VCE has demonstrated a high diagnostic yield.[84] When performed for suspected small bowel bleeding, repeat VCE demonstrated a diagnostic yield of 45.8% to 73.2% after initial negative capsule study.[85,86]

SUMMARY

VCE and DAE are complementary technologies with similar diagnostic yields. Capsule endoscopy as a prelude to DAE in suspected small bowel bleeding is less invasive, has good patient acceptance, and high diagnostic yield, and guides DAE or surgical approach to therapy. For VCE to be effective before DAE, competence in capsule reading is crucial. Familiarity with the capabilities of VCE and its limitations minimizes the risk for overreading normal or clinically insignificant findings and reduces the potential for missed lesions. Future work is required to improve the accuracy of VCE reading, lesion localization, and the development of a steerable device that would allow for tissue sampling and therapy.

CLINICS CARE POINTS

- Video capsule endoscopy is the recommended initial diagnostic test in suspected small bowel bleeding with a high patient acceptance and diagnostic accuracy.
- Timing of video capsule endoscopy performance and subsequent device-assisted enteroscopy is critical in an overt bleeding presentation.
- Early use of video capsule endoscopy in the setting of gastrointestinal bleeding allows for a directed approach to therapeutic endoscopy.

ACKNOWLEDGMENTS

None.

SUPPLEMENTARY DATA

Supplementary data related to this article can be found online at https://doi.org/10.1016/j.giec.2020.12.008.

REFERENCES

1. May A, Nachbar L, Schneider M, et al. Prospective comparison of push enteroscopy and push-and-pull enteroscopy in patients with suspected small-bowel bleeding. Am J Gastroenterol 2006;101(9):2016–24.
2. Yamamoto H, Sekine Y, Sato Y, et al. Total enteroscopy with a nonsurgical steerable double-balloon method. Gastrointest Endosc 2001;53(2):216–20.
3. Semrad CE. Small bowel enteroscopy: territory conquered, future horizons. Curr Opin Gastroenterol 2009;25(2):110–5.
4. May A, Farber M, Aschmoneit I, et al. Prospective multicenter trial comparing push-and-pull enteroscopy with the single- and double-balloon techniques in patients with small-bowel disorders. Am J Gastroenterol 2010;105(3):575–81.
5. Akerman PA, Agrawal D, Chen W, et al. Spiral enteroscopy: a novel method of enteroscopy by using the Endo-Ease Discovery SB overtube and a pediatric colonoscope. Gastrointest Endosc 2009;69(2):327–32.
6. Judah JR, Draganov PV, Lam Y, et al. Spiral enteroscopy is safe and effective for an elderly United States population of patients with numerous comorbidities. Clin Gastroenterol Hepatol 2010;8(7):572–6.
7. Khashab MA, Lennon AM, Dunbar KB, et al. A comparative evaluation of single-balloon enteroscopy and spiral enteroscopy for patients with mid-gut disorders. Gastrointest Endosc 2010;72(4):766–72.

8. Ali R, Wild D, Shieh F, et al. Deep enteroscopy with a conventional colonoscope: initial multicenter study by using a through-the-scope balloon catheter system. Gastrointest Endosc 2015;82(5):855–60.

9. Ross AS, Dye C, Prachand VN. Laparoscopic-assisted double-balloon enteroscopy for small-bowel polyp surveillance and treatment in patients with Peutz-Jeghers syndrome. Gastrointest Endosc 2006;64(6):984–8.

10. Johnston SJ, Jones PF, Kyle J, et al. Epidemiology and course of gastrointestinal haemorrhage in North-east Scotland. Br Med J 1973;3(5882):655–60.

11. Raju GS, Gerson L, Das A, et al. American Gastroenterological Association (AGA) Institute technical review on obscure gastrointestinal bleeding. Gastroenterology 2007;133(5):1697–717.

12. Spiller RC, Parkins RA. Recurrent gastrointestinal bleeding of obscure origin: report of 17 cases and a guide to logical management. Br J Surg 1983;70(8): 489–93.

13. Igawa A, Oka S, Tanaka S, et al. Major predictors and management of small-bowel angioectasia. BMC Gastroenterol 2015;15:108.

14. Jackson CS, Gerson LB. Management of gastrointestinal angiodysplastic lesions (GIADs): a systematic review and meta-analysis. Am J Gastroenterol 2014; 109(4):474–83 [quiz: 84].

15. Enns RA, Hookey L, Armstrong D, et al. Clinical practice guidelines for the use of video capsule endoscopy. Gastroenterology 2017;152(3):497–514.

16. Cook JD. Diagnosis and management of iron-deficiency anaemia. Best Pract Res Clin Haematol 2005;18(2):319–32.

17. Lee MW, Pourmorady JS, Laine L. Use of fecal occult blood testing as a diagnostic tool for clinical indications: a systematic review and meta-analysis. Am J Gastroenterol 2020;115(5):662–70.

18. Goddard AF, James MW, McIntyre AS, et al. Guidelines for the management of iron deficiency anaemia. Gut 2011;60(10):1309–16.

19. Endo H, Kato T, Sakai E, et al. Is a fecal occult blood test a useful tool for judging whether to perform capsule endoscopy in low-dose aspirin users with negative colonoscopy and esophagogastroduodenoscopy? J Gastroenterol 2017;52(2): 194–202.

20. Kobayashi Y, Watabe H, Yamada A, et al. Impact of fecal occult blood on obscure gastrointestinal bleeding: observational study. World J Gastroenterol 2015;21(1): 326–32.

21. Shiotani A, Tarumi K, Honda K, et al. Application of fecal hemoglobin-haptoglobin complex testing for small bowel lesions. Scand J Gastroenterol 2014;49(5): 539–44.

22. Segarajasingam DS, Hanley SC, Barkun AN, et al. Randomized controlled trial comparing outcomes of video capsule endoscopy with push enteroscopy in obscure gastrointestinal bleeding. Can J Gastroenterol Hepatol 2015;29(2): 85–90.

23. Hadithi M, Heine GD, Jacobs MA, et al. A prospective study comparing video capsule endoscopy with double-balloon enteroscopy in patients with obscure gastrointestinal bleeding. Am J Gastroenterol 2006;101(1):52–7.

24. Pasha SF, Leighton JA, Das A, et al. Double-balloon enteroscopy and capsule endoscopy have comparable diagnostic yield in small-bowel disease: a meta-analysis. Clin Gastroenterol Hepatol 2008;6(6):671–6.

25. Arakawa D, Ohmiya N, Nakamura M, et al. Outcome after enteroscopy for patients with obscure GI bleeding: diagnostic comparison between double-

balloon endoscopy and videocapsule endoscopy. Gastrointest Endosc 2009; 69(4):866–74.

26. Law R, Varayil JE, WongKeeSong LM, et al. Assessment of multi-modality evaluations of obscure gastrointestinal bleeding. World J Gastroenterol 2017;23(4): 614–21.

27. Gerson L, Kamal A. Cost-effectiveness analysis of management strategies for obscure GI bleeding. Gastrointest Endosc 2008;68(5):920–36.

28. Jawaid S, Marya NB, Hicks M, et al. Prospective cost analysis of early video capsule endoscopy versus standard of care in non-hematemesis gastrointestinal bleeding: a non-inferiority study. J Med Econ 2020;23(1):10–6.

29. Meltzer AC, Ward MJ, Gralnek IM, et al. The cost-effectiveness analysis of video capsule endoscopy compared to other strategies to manage acute upper gastrointestinal hemorrhage in the ED. Am J Emerg Med 2014;32(8):823–32.

30. Meltzer AC, Ali MA, Kresiberg RB, et al. Video capsule endoscopy in the emergency department: a prospective study of acute upper gastrointestinal hemorrhage. Ann Emerg Med 2013;61(4):438–43.e1.

31. Gay G, Delvaux M, Fassler I. Outcome of capsule endoscopy in determining indication and route for push-and-pull enteroscopy. Endoscopy 2006;38(1):49–58.

32. Li X, Chen H, Dai J, et al. Predictive role of capsule endoscopy on the insertion route of double-balloon enteroscopy. Endoscopy 2009;41(9):762–6.

33. Nakamura M, Ohmiya N, Shirai O, et al. Route selection for double-balloon endoscopy, based on capsule transit time, in obscure gastrointestinal bleeding. J Gastroenterol 2010;45(6):592–9.

34. Gerson LB, Fidler JL, Cave DR, et al. ACG Clinical Guideline: diagnosis and management of small bowel bleeding. Am J Gastroenterol 2015;110(9):1265–87 [quiz: 88].

35. Vlachogiannakos J, Papaxoinis K, Viazis N, et al. Bleeding lesions within reach of conventional endoscopy in capsule endoscopy examinations for obscure gastrointestinal bleeding: is repeating endoscopy economically feasible? Dig Dis Sci 2011;56(6):1763–8.

36. Lepileur L, Dray X, Antonietti M, et al. Factors associated with diagnosis of obscure gastrointestinal bleeding by video capsule enteroscopy. Clin Gastroenterol Hepatol 2012;10(12):1376–80.

37. Robinson CA, Jackson C, Condon D, et al. Impact of inpatient status and gender on small-bowel capsule endoscopy findings. Gastrointest Endosc 2011;74(5): 1061–6.

38. Singh A, Marshall C, Chaudhuri B, et al. Timing of video capsule endoscopy relative to overt obscure GI bleeding: implications from a retrospective study. Gastrointest Endosc 2013;77(5):761–6.

39. Pennazio M, Santucci R, Rondonotti E, et al. Outcome of patients with obscure gastrointestinal bleeding after capsule endoscopy: report of 100 consecutive cases. Gastroenterology 2004;126(3):643–53.

40. Nennstiel S, Machanek A, von Delius S, et al. Predictors and characteristics of angioectasias in patients with obscure gastrointestinal bleeding identified by video capsule endoscopy. United European Gastroenterol J 2017;5(8):1129–35.

41. Papadopoulos AA, Triantafyllou K, Kalantzis C, et al. Effects of ageing on small bowel video-capsule endoscopy examination. Am J Gastroenterol 2008; 103(10):2474–80.

42. Scaglione G, Russo F, Franco MR, et al. Age and video capsule endoscopy in obscure gastrointestinal bleeding: a prospective study on hospitalized patients. Dig Dis Sci 2011;56(4):1188–93.

43. Song JH, Hong SN, Kyung Chang D, et al. The etiology of potential small-bowel bleeding depending on patient's age and gender. United European Gastroenterol J 2018;6(8):1169–78.

44. Cho KM, Park SY, Chung JO, et al. Risk factors for small bowel bleeding in chronic nonsteroidal anti-inflammatory drug users. J Dig Dis 2015;16(9):499–504.

45. Tziatzios G, Gkolfakis P, Papanikolaou IS, et al. Antithrombotic treatment is associated with small-bowel video capsule endoscopy positive findings in obscure gastrointestinal bleeding: a systematic review and meta-analysis. Dig Dis Sci 2019;64(1):15–24.

46. Van Weyenberg SJ, Van Turenhout ST, Jacobs MA, et al. Video capsule endoscopy for previous overt obscure gastrointestinal bleeding in patients using antithrombotic drugs. Dig Endosc 2012;24(4):247–54.

47. Schlag C, Menzel C, Nennstiel S, et al. Emergency video capsule endoscopy in patients with acute severe GI bleeding and negative upper endoscopy results. Gastrointest Endosc 2015;81(4):889–95.

48. Lecleire S, Iwanicki-Caron I, Di-Fiore A, et al. Yield and impact of emergency capsule enteroscopy in severe obscure-overt gastrointestinal bleeding. Endoscopy 2012;44(4):337–42.

49. Marya NB, Jawaid S, Foley A, et al. A randomized controlled trial comparing efficacy of early video capsule endoscopy with standard of care in the approach to nonhematemesis GI bleeding (with videos). Gastrointest Endosc 2019;89(1):33–43.e4.

50. Pennazio M, Rondonotti E, Koulaouzidis A. Small bowel capsule endoscopy: normal findings and normal variants of the small bowel. Gastrointest Endosc Clin N Am 2017;27(1):29–50.

51. Rondonotti E, Pennazio M, Toth E, et al. Small-bowel neoplasms in patients undergoing video capsule endoscopy: a multicenter European study. Endoscopy 2008;40(6):488–95.

52. Lim YJ, Lee OY, Jeen YT, et al. Indications for detection, completion, and retention rates of small bowel capsule endoscopy based on the 10-year data from the Korean Capsule Endoscopy Registry. Clin Endosc 2015;48(5):399–404.

53. Cheung DY, Kim JS, Shim KN, et al. The usefulness of capsule endoscopy for small bowel tumors. Clin Endosc 2016;49(1):21–5.

54. Goodman MT, Matsuno RK, Shvetsov YB. Racial and ethnic variation in the incidence of small-bowel cancer subtypes in the United States, 1995-2008. Dis Colon Rectum 2013;56(4):441–8.

55. van Leerdam ME, Roos VH, van Hooft JE, et al. Endoscopic management of polyposis syndromes: European Society of Gastrointestinal Endoscopy (ESGE) Guideline. Endoscopy 2019;51(9):877–95.

56. Yang J, Gurudu SR, Koptiuch C, et al. American Society for Gastrointestinal Endoscopy guideline on the role of endoscopy in familial adenomatous polyposis syndromes. Gastrointest Endosc 2020;91(5):963–82.e2.

57. Ross A, Mehdizadeh S, Tokar J, et al. Double balloon enteroscopy detects small bowel mass lesions missed by capsule endoscopy. Dig Dis Sci 2008;53(8):2140–3.

58. Lewis BS, Eisen GM, Friedman S. A pooled analysis to evaluate results of capsule endoscopy trials. Endoscopy 2005;37(10):960–5.

59. Zagorowicz ES, Pietrzak AM, Wronska E, et al. Small bowel tumors detected and missed during capsule endoscopy: single center experience. World J Gastroenterol 2013;19(47):9043–8.

60. Limsrivilai J, Srisajjakul S, Pongprasobchai S, et al. A prospective blinded comparison of video capsule endoscopy versus computed tomography enterography in potential small bowel bleeding: clinical utility of computed tomography enterography. J Clin Gastroenterol 2017;51(7):611–8.

61. Cave D, Legnani P, de Franchis R, et al. ICCE consensus for capsule retention. Endoscopy 2005;37(10):1065–7.

62. Al-Bawardy B, Locke G, Huprich JE, et al. Retained capsule endoscopy in a large tertiary care academic practice and radiologic predictors of retention. Inflamm Bowel Dis 2015;21(9):2158–64.

63. Cheifetz AS, Kornbluth AA, Legnani P, et al. The risk of retention of the capsule endoscope in patients with known or suspected Crohn's disease. Am J Gastroenterol 2006;101(10):2218–22.

64. Li F, Gurudu SR, De Petris G, et al. Retention of the capsule endoscope: a single-center experience of 1000 capsule endoscopy procedures. Gastrointest Endosc 2008;68(1):174–80.

65. Cheifetz AS, Lewis BS. Capsule endoscopy retention: is it a complication? J Clin Gastroenterol 2006;40(8):688–91.

66. Rozendorn N, Klang E, Lahat A, et al. Prediction of patency capsule retention in known Crohn's disease patients by using magnetic resonance imaging. Gastrointest Endosc 2016;83(1):182–7.

67. Herrerias JM, Leighton JA, Costamagna G, et al. Agile patency system eliminates risk of capsule retention in patients with known intestinal strictures who undergo capsule endoscopy. Gastrointest Endosc 2008;67(6):902–9.

68. Van Weyenberg SJ, Van Turenhout ST, Bouma G, et al. Double-balloon endoscopy as the primary method for small-bowel video capsule endoscope retrieval. Gastrointest Endosc 2010;71(3):535–41.

69. Gao Y, Xin L, Wang YX, et al. Double-balloon enteroscopy for retrieving retained small-bowel video capsule endoscopes: a systematic review. Scand J Gastroenterol 2020;55(1):105–13.

70. Gerson LB, Batenic MA, Newsom SL, et al. Long-term outcomes after double-balloon enteroscopy for obscure gastrointestinal bleeding. Clin Gastroenterol Hepatol 2009;7(6):664–9.

71. Rahmi G, Samaha E, Vahedi K, et al. Long-term follow-up of patients undergoing capsule and double-balloon enteroscopy for identification and treatment of small-bowel vascular lesions: a prospective, multicenter study. Endoscopy 2014;46(7):591–7.

72. Samaha E, Rahmi G, Landi B, et al. Long-term outcome of patients treated with double balloon enteroscopy for small bowel vascular lesions. Am J Gastroenterol 2012;107(2):240–6.

73. Laine L, Sahota A, Shah A. Does capsule endoscopy improve outcomes in obscure gastrointestinal bleeding? Randomized trial versus dedicated small bowel radiography. Gastroenterology 2010;138(5):1673–80.e1 [quiz: e11–2].

74. Katsinelos P, Lazaraki G, Gkagkalis A, et al. The role of capsule endoscopy in the evaluation and treatment of obscure-overt gastrointestinal bleeding during daily clinical practice: a prospective multicenter study. Scand J Gastroenterol 2014;49(7):862–70.

75. Shinozaki S, Yamamoto H, Yano T, et al. Favorable long-term outcomes of repeat endotherapy for small-intestine vascular lesions by double-balloon endoscopy. Gastrointest Endosc 2014;80(1):112–7.

76. Min YW, Kim JS, Jeon SW, et al. Long-term outcome of capsule endoscopy in obscure gastrointestinal bleeding: a nationwide analysis. Endoscopy 2014; 46(1):59–65.
77. Niikura R, Yamada A, Nagata N, et al. New predictive model of rebleeding during follow-up of patents with obscure gastrointestinal bleeding: a multicenter cohort study. J Gastroenterol Hepatol 2016;31(4):752–60.
78. de Sousa Magalhães R, Cúrdia Gonçalves T, Rosa B, et al. RHEMITT score: predicting the risk of rebleeding for patients with mid-gastrointestinal bleeding submitted to small bowel capsule endoscopy. Dig Dis 2020;38(4):299–309.
79. Silva JC, Pinho R, Ponte A, et al. Predicting the risk of rebleeding after capsule endoscopy in obscure gastrointestinal bleeding - External validation of the RHEMITT Score. Dig Dis 2020;8(10):000509986.
80. Albert JG, Schülbe R, Hahn L, et al. Impact of capsule endoscopy on outcome in mid-intestinal bleeding: a multicentre cohort study in 285 patients. Eur J Gastroenterol Hepatol 2008;20(10):971–7.
81. Lai LH, Wong GL, Chow DK, et al. Long-term follow-up of patients with obscure gastrointestinal bleeding after negative capsule endoscopy. Am J Gastroenterol 2006;101(6):1224–8.
82. Yung DE, Koulaouzidis A, Avni T, et al. Clinical outcomes of negative small-bowel capsule endoscopy for small-bowel bleeding: a systematic review and meta-analysis. Gastrointest Endosc 2017;85(2):305–17.e2.
83. Lorenceau-Savale C, Ben-Soussan E, Ramirez S, et al. Outcome of patients with obscure gastrointestinal bleeding after negative capsule endoscopy: results of a one-year follow-up study. Gastroenterol Clin Biol 2010;34(11):606–11.
84. Jones BH, Fleischer DE, Sharma VK, et al. Yield of repeat wireless video capsule endoscopy in patients with obscure gastrointestinal bleeding. Am J Gastroenterol 2005;100(5):1058–64.
85. Otani K, Watanabe T, Shimada S, et al. Usefulness of small bowel reexamination in obscure gastrointestinal bleeding patients with negative capsule endoscopy findings: comparison of repeat capsule endoscopy and double-balloon enteroscopy. United European Gastroenterol J 2018;6(6):879–87.
86. Robertson AR, Yung DE, Douglas S, et al. Repeat capsule endoscopy in suspected gastrointestinal bleeding. Scand J Gastroenterol 2019;54(5):656–61.

Role of Capsule Endoscopy in Inflammatory Bowel Disease

Josiah D. McCain, MD, Shabana F. Pasha, MD,
Jonathan A. Leighton, MD*

KEYWORDS

- Crohn disease • Ulcerative colitis • Capsule endoscopy

KEY POINTS

- Capsule endoscopy (CE) is highly sensitive, but not specific, for mucosal inflammation.
- CE in inflammatory bowel disease is most useful when ileocolonoscopy is negative, especially if cross-sectional imaging is also negative.
- The benefits of CE in established Crohn disease (CD) include identifying location of disease, rating severity, and monitoring response to therapy or treat to target.
- The benefit of CE in suspected CD is mainly as a tool to exclude the diagnosis.
- The major complication of CE in CD is capsule retention, but the risk can be significantly reduced by performance of patency capsule or cross-sectional small bowel imaging in established CD.

 Video content accompanies this article at http://www.giendo.theclinics.com.

INTRODUCTION

Capsule endoscopy (CE) has been extensively studied in the diagnosis and management of inflammatory bowel disease (IBD). Studies suggest that it has a role in suspected and established Crohn disease (CD). There is also emerging evidence that it could play a role in ulcerative colitis (UC) but support for this is currently limited. The biggest advantage of CE is that it enables visualization of the entire length of the small bowel and is less invasive than standard fiberoptic endoscopes (Video 1). As with any relatively new technology, it is an evolving modality. With the development of colon capsule endoscopy (CCE) and the pan-enteric capsule endoscopy (PCE), direct visualization of both small bowel and colon can be achieved in both CD and

Division of Gastroenterology and Hepatology, Mayo Clinic, 13400 East Shea Boulevard, Scottsdale, AZ 85259, USA
* Corresponding author.
E-mail address: Leighton.jonathan@mayo.edu

Gastrointest Endoscopy Clin N Am 31 (2021) 345–361
https://doi.org/10.1016/j.giec.2020.12.004
1052-5157/21/© 2020 Elsevier Inc. All rights reserved.
giendo.theclinics.com

UC. Understanding the strengths and limitations of CE in the diagnosis and management of IBD, as well as the current trends and future directions, is an important component of treating patients with these disorders.

CROHN DISEASE

CD is an idiopathic IBD that can occur anywhere along the gastrointestinal tract, and is characterized by mucosal or transmural inflammation. Any evaluation of a patient with CD must include the gastrointestinal mucosa. This is traditionally performed using colonoscopy with terminal ileal inspection. Upper endoscopy may also be indicated in pediatrics and those adults with upper tract symptoms. Up to 30% of patients with CD have disease that is confined to the small bowel.[1]

There are several potential roles for CE in the evaluation of patients with CD. These roles will vary based on whether or not the patient has suspected versus established CD. In patients whose small bowel CD is confined to areas proximal to the terminal ileum, traditional ileocolonoscopy provides a challenge in the generation of a timely diagnosis.[2] In this subset of patients especially, supplemental, nontraditional means of visualizing the bowel may be necessary both to provide diagnosis and to survey active disease.

Capsule Endoscopy Compared with Other Diagnostic Modalities

Commonly, patients with early or mild CD will manifest mucosal disruption that can be subtle and diagnostically elusive. These small abnormalities may be missed by diagnostic modalities that do not directly visualize the mucosa, such as cross-sectional imaging studies. In these patients, CE carries a distinct advantage. In addition to its ability to directly visualize the small bowel inaccessible by traditional ileocolonoscopy, CE can detect subtle mucosal changes that are easily missed on cross-sectional imaging (**Fig. 1**). In a meta-analysis that compared CE with other modalities in the detection of superficial mucosal disruption, CE had a better diagnostic yield than all others. CE exceeded the detection ability of small bowel follow-through by 63% versus 23% ($P<.001$), it exceeded ileocolonoscopy by 61% versus 46% ($P = .02$), and by 69% versus 30% ($P = .001$) when compared with computed tomography enterography (CTE).[3] In a more recent comparison, a meta-analysis of CE performance against other diagnostic modalities validated its usefulness. In analysis of that data, CE had higher incremental diagnostic yields in nonstricturing CD over push enteroscopy at 42%, CTE at 39%, small bowel radiographs at 37%, and ileoscopy at 15%.[4] Overall, the diagnostic yield of CE in CD ranges from 43% to 71%, and CE is shown to be superior to imaging both in diagnosis of suspected CD and in the evaluation of established disease.[5–8] In a comparison study with magnetic resonance enterography (MRE), 30 patients with suspected or known CD underwent CE, MRE, and ileocolonoscopy. In that study, CE was more sensitive than MRE for detecting small bowel inflammatory changes (80% vs 76%), less specific (88% vs 90%), and more accurate overall (90% vs 83%).[9] Another study that retrospectively compared MRE to CE findings in 47 patients with known or suspected CD found CE was superior in detecting small bowel lesions, detecting abnormalities in 76.6% of patients versus 44.7% by MRE ($P = .001$).[10] A prospective, blinded comparison trail of CE, CTE, ileocolonoscopy, and barium small bowel radiography demonstrated sensitivities of 83%, 83%, 74%, and 65%, respectively. However, it also established a specificity of 53%, significantly lower than the other 3 modalities ($P<.05$).[11] Another study prospectively comparing CTE, MRE, and CE in 93 patients with suspected or newly diagnosed CD, cited a sensitivity of CE for detecting active CD lesions in the terminal ileum of 100% and a

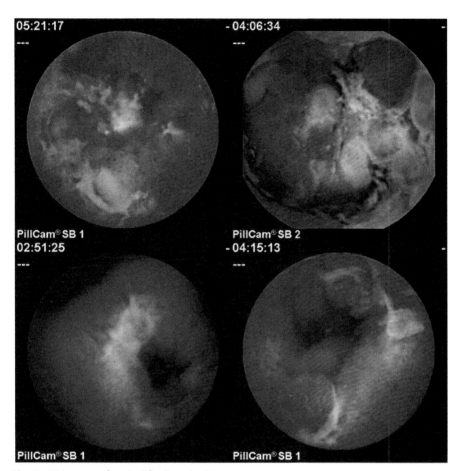

Fig. 1. CE images of typical findings in CD.

specificity of 91%. This is compared with sensitivity and specificity of MRE at 81% and 86% and of CTE at 76% and 85%, respectively. In the same study, CE detected proximal lesions in 18 of the patients, with MRE detecting lesions in 2 and CTE in 6 patients only (P<.05).[12]

Suspected Crohn Disease

In patients with suspected CD, the most appropriate first evaluation remains ileocolonoscopy in most cases. A negative ileocolonoscopy, however, does not exclude the possibility of more proximal small bowel CD. There are data to suggest that CE can be a useful tool in this set of patients. In the diagnosis of small bowel CD, CE has been demonstrated to have a sensitivity of 93% and a specificity of 84%.[13] The utility of CE, and its diagnostic yield, can be further enhanced when coupled with other markers of disease. Fecal calprotectin is one such tool. Fecal calprotectin has been proven a useful indicator that allows for enrichment of patient selection for CE in evaluation of suspected CD,[14–16] potentially reducing false positive results. As the low specificity of CE in the small bowel remains its major weakness, pairing it with markers such as fecal calprotectin may be an important strategy in enhancing its overall performance. However, because of its reported low specificity, CE is perhaps most valuable when negative in the evaluation CD. In ruling out CD, CE has a demonstrated negative predictive value of 96%.[17]

As we have highlighted, CE has a specificity that is relatively low. This is an important limitation that should be understood if it is to be used effectively. As a highly sensitive tool, CE may detect other inflammatory lesions of the small bowel, and not all of these will be clinically relevant for the patient or specific to the diagnosis of CD. Asymptomatic mucosal lesions that have no clinical significance may be observed in many patients undergoing CE. Nonsteroidal anti-inflammatory drugs (NSAIDs) are known to cause small bowel stenoses called NSAID enteropathy or Diaphragm Disease that can mimic CD on visual inspection.[18] NSAIDs can also cause mucosal erosions and ulcerations. It is important, therefore, that patients undergoing CE be instructed to avoid NSAIDs for at least 4 weeks prior to minimize false positive test results. Infection, autoimmune disease, radiation, immunodeficiency, ischemia, celiac disease, and other drug-induced injuries in addition to NSAID enteropathy also can cause abnormalities that may be difficult to differentiate from CD on CE.[19,20]

In summary, CE maintains a high negative predictive value and a low specificity for diagnosis of CD. It is therefore most useful as a tool for exclusion of CD, rather than a confirmation of diagnosis. **Fig. 2** demonstrates an algorithm highlighting the role of CE in the evaluation of patients with suspected CD.

Established Crohn Disease

CE has the potential to play a significant role in the management of patients with established CD. CE can provide detailed information that cross-sectional imaging and ileocolonoscopy may fail to yield, and therefore provides useful information in the monitoring of disease activity.

Assessing distribution and activity of disease

Assessing the activity of disease, and its distribution are key components in the management of CD. This is particularly true in the new era of "treat to target" strategies, wherein mucosal healing is the hallmark of successful therapy.[21] To this end, the role of CE in patients with established CD is an area that continues to evolve. For CE to be consistently effective, its use must be standardized, and tools such as scoring systems of disease ought to be applied. Two such tools, the Lewis Score[22] and the Capsule Endoscopy Crohn's Disease Activity Index (CECDAI),[23] have been suggested. The 2 are similar in that they measure extent and severity of inflammation

Suggested evaluation of patients with suspected CD

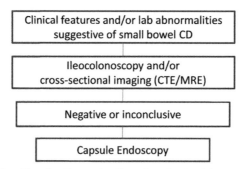

Fig. 2. Suggested algorithm for the evaluation of patients with suspected CD using CE.

and presence of strictures. They differ mainly in how these are measured and scored. Various studies have undertaken to compare, analyze, and/or incorporate these scores into clinical practice, and data suggest that they may be useful in predicting relapse or hospitalization rates in patients with CD.[24–26] Nonetheless, larger prospective studies are needed for validation and broader incorporation of a standardized grading system. As yet, neither the Lewis Score, nor the CECDAI have found their way into common clinical practice.[27]

One area in which CE evaluation can be helpful is in the patient with overlapping CD and irritable bowel syndrome. In this population of patients, CE can be useful for distinguishing the level of symptoms attributable to CD activity. For example, CE can act as a tool for assessing small bowel disease in the patient with CD who may not be showing a clinical response to medications in the setting of normal ileocolonoscopy and/or cross-sectional imaging.[28–31]

One study analyzed 108 patients with known CD with CE and found jejunal lesions in 56% of them. It also established that the presence of jejunal lesions associates with increased risk of relapsing disease.[32]

Findings on CE have been shown to change management in a substantial number of cases of known CD. The cost-benefit ratio of CE analysis in patients with known CD has not, as yet, defined a clear role in its impact on clinical outcomes and decreasing health care costs.[33]

Postoperative recurrence

The postoperative assessment of patients with CD can be important in determining long-term management of the disease. In such cases, CE may be of benefit, especially if the area of involvement is not accessible via ileocolonoscopy. However, there is some disagreement in the utility of CE in this role. In evaluation of the neoterminal ileum after ileocolonic resection, CE has been cited as having a lower sensitivity than ileocolonoscopy in the detection of lesions proximal to the surgical anastomosis.[34] Some investigators, in contrast, suggest that CE provides a significant increase in the diagnostic yield of mucosal disruptions proximal to the anastomosis; particularly where they may be out of reach of an endoscope.[34,35] In current practice, ileocolonoscopy remains the generally accepted diagnostic procedure of choice in the postoperative evaluation of CD. Still, there remains a subset of postoperative patients wherein the surgical area is not reachable via endoscopic means. It may be that CE is the best choice for evaluation of postoperative occurrence in these patients.

Inflammatory bowel disease–undefined

The term IBD-undefined (IBDU) refers to inflammatory colitis wherein the specific diagnosis of UC versus CD cannot be made. This distinction is important, as there is a significant difference in surgical management of patients with UC and Crohn colitis. In these patients, an evaluation of the small bowel may provide a diagnosis of CD. There are studies that have shown that CE can detect small bowel lesions consistent with CD in 29% to 40% of patients, although these have been small and uncontrolled studies.[3,36,37] Additional data show the ability of CE to classify lesions in the small bowel, and provide diagnostic information for clinicians in these types of patients. These studies show that CE is a useful tool in diagnosing CD in a patient with IBDU. These studies have specifically demonstrated that CE can detect previously unknown lesions in patients with IBDU and UC with atypical features that may alter the diagnosis.[38–41] A negative result, although not as useful in terms of diagnosis, can still effectively rule out small bowel involvement, owing to the high sensitivity of CE. This can aid in further clarifying the clinical picture in the patient with IBDU.

Mucosal healing and treat to target

As mentioned previously, the assessment of mucosal healing in the patient with established CD is an important clinical benchmark for the physician, and one that can be assisted by CE. Mucosal healing is one of the most objective methods by means of which response to medical therapy can be observed, measured, and documented. Clinical improvement, too, is helpful in monitoring CD and therapy response. However, assessment of symptoms can be a poor indication and does not consistently correlate with severity and extent of disease.[21] As we have emphasized throughout this article, CE can detect very subtle mucosal abnormalities that other, less sensitive modalities might miss.[27] It is therefore true that the use of CE in monitoring of disease, and of medication response, can and will change medical therapies and strategies and influence disease outcomes. It has been documented, in fact, that CE has changed therapy in a significant number of patient cases.[33] Additional evidence has shown that signs of mucosal healing in the small bowel after 1 year of treatment for IBD is predictive of reduced activity in the future, and associates with a decreased need for subsequent treatment.[42] When mucosal healing is emphasized as a primary endpoint of CD therapy, CE can facilitate the monitoring of disease state and thus guide management.[43] Future studies are needed to definitively characterize the relationship between the mucosal healing demonstrated on CE, and patient-determined clinical response to therapy. However, it is reasonable, and forward-thinking, to consider that CE may have a unique and useful role to play in the surveillance of patients with small bowel CD.

Fig. 3 demonstrates an algorithm highlighting the role of CE in the evaluation of patients with established CD.

Mimics of Crohn Disease on Capsule Endoscopy

Nonsteroidal anti-inflammatory drug–associated injury

NSAIDs can affect the gastrointestinal tract in several detrimental fashions. Mucosal ulcerations, acute and chronic gastrointestinal hemorrhage, hypoalbuminemia, malabsorption, obstruction, and the characteristic diaphragms can all be caused by NSAID usage.[44]

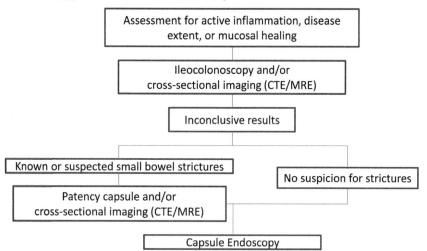

Suggested evaluation of patients with established CD

Fig. 3. Suggested algorithm for the evaluation of patients with established CD using CE.

In detection of NSAID-induced mucosal injury, CE can be used as a sensitive diagnostic tool. The mucosal disruptions caused by NSAIDs can be picked up by CE up to 68% of the time.[44,45] A study comparing the CE findings of 21 chronic NSAID users with 20 controls found mucosal disruptions in the small bowel (red spots, erosions, or ulcers) in 71% of the cases in comparison with 10% of the controls.[46] A prospective study assigned patients to daily NSAIDs or placebo and analyzed them with baseline and interval CE studies. The investigators found that mucosal breaks developed in the 2 groups of patients taking daily NSAIDs at a rate of 55% and 16%, whereas in the group taking placebo, only 7% developed any signs of damage.[18]

NSAID enteropathy, or diaphragm disease, is characterized by thin, circumferential membranes or stenoses in the small bowel (**Fig. 4**). The major complications of diaphragm disease are obstruction and iron deficiency anemia, although most NSAID-induced injury is likely subclinical. The stricturing lesions can occur as a single membrane or as multiple along the small bowel, usually in the mid to distal ileum, and typically occur after years of NSAID use.[44,47]

Diaphragm disease is difficult to diagnose. Typically, upper endoscopy and ileocolonoscopy will yield a normal result. Neither does cross-sectional imaging consistently

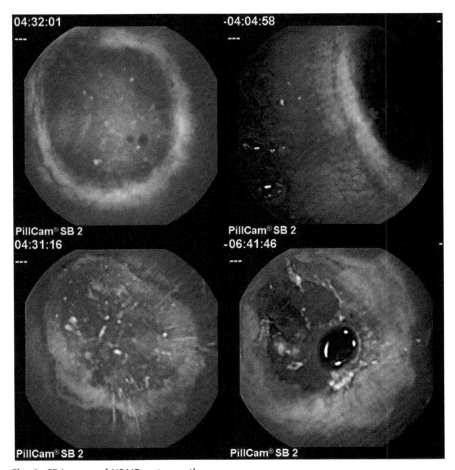

Fig. 4. CE images of NSAID enteropathy.

provide a diagnosis.[47] Often, the appearance of diaphragms in the small bowel have been misinterpreted as plicae circularis on computed tomography (CT), MRI, or small bowel follow-through.[48] Increasing awareness of the disease, however, and the use of multiphase or multisequence imaging via CTE or MRE may help in the diagnosis. Deep enteroscopy has been the modality of choice in diagnosing diaphragm disease, as it provides direct visualization of the lesions themselves. Deep enteroscopy also carries the benefit of possible therapeutic intervention on symptomatic lesions. Because the muscularis propria is not compromised in the diaphragms, dilation of the strictures via endoscopy seems to carry a low perforation risk.[49]

The major adverse event of CE in NSAID enteropathy is capsule retention. In a study of 1000 CE procedures, retention occurred in 14 cases. In 11 of those cases (79%), NSAID enteropathy was the culprit. In each of those patients, radiologic studies were negative.[50] Because much of NSAID-induced injury is asymptomatic, adequate screening can be challenging. A thorough history and medication reconciliation are imperative before submitting a patient for CE. Patients in whom NSAID enteropathy is suspected should undergo small bowel imaging or patency capsule before CE, to reduce risk of capsule retention.[50]

Other inflammatory conditions of the bowel

Case reports have been published wherein CE aided in the diagnosis of radiation enteritis in patients with anemia and melena.[51–53] Moreover, one pilot study enrolled 15 patients with chronic abdominal pain or anemia after radiation therapy for pancreatic cancer to test the feasibility of using CE for diagnosis of radiation enteritis. The investigators found lesions suspicious for radiation enteritis in 9 patients (60%) with no episodes of capsule retention. The most common findings on CE were erythema and congested mucosa.[54]

Eosinophilic enteritis is a rare disease in the class of the gastrointestinal eosinophilic disorders. Definitive diagnosis is made via histologic examination, but endoscopic visualization can be suggestive. Findings of eosinophilic enteritis on CE may be nonspecific, but can include erythema, congestion, erosions, ulcerations, and stenotic lesions.[55–57]

Autoimmune enteropathy is another rare inflammatory disease of the gastrointestinal tract characterized by severe villous atrophy of the small bowel in the absence of dietary triggers. This results in a spruelike illness causing diarrhea, malabsorption, and weight loss. Although histologic analysis is necessary for diagnosis, CE can provide typical endoscopic findings. These include blunted villi, scalloping, fissures, and aphthous ulcers.[58,59]

ULCERATIVE COLITIS

UC is chronic disease of the colon and rectum that is characterized by diffuse confluent mucosal inflammation. When compared with CD, there is considerably less published research regarding the use of CE in UC. The primary role for CE in these patients may be when the diagnosis of UC is in question.

Direct visualization of the epithelial surface of the colon and the terminal ileum is an important part of the diagnosis and management of UC. Most often, this is achieved through ileocolonoscopy. CCE may have a role in certain patients and scenarios, and recent comparison studies between the 2 modalities have helped to clarify those. One such study of 29 pediatric patients with UC cited a sensitivity of 96% and a specificity of 100% for CCE.[60] Another study of 100 patients with UC found that CCE had a sensitivity of 89% and a specificity of 75%.[61] In a more recent prospective study, CCE showed a sensitivity of 97% to detect mucosal inflammation, and displayed substantial agreement with colonoscopy findings using the Mayo endoscopic score and the Ulcerative Colitis Endoscopic Index of Severity with ICCs of 0.69 and 0.64, respectively. In addition, CCE was both better tolerated and preferred by patients over colonoscopy.[62]

The precise role of CCE in UC remains to be defined. As in CD, mucosal healing is a primary endpoint of UC management, making endoscopic surveillance a necessary component of patient care.[21] Strengths of CCE in UC seem to be its tolerability and sensitivity. Compared with standard ileocolonoscopy, it is noninvasive and reduces time away from work for patients. However, CCE requires an extensive bowel prep with boosters, and unlike ileocolonoscopy it does not allow for tissue sampling. Questions regarding the cost-effectiveness of CCE compared with ileocolonoscopy have yet to be answered, and more research needs to be done before the true diagnostic accuracy of this test can be understood.

COLON CAPSULE ENDOSCOPY AND PAN-ENTERIC CAPSULES

CCE is a relatively new area of CE wherein preliminary studies have evaluated its role in both CD and UC. One such study prospectively evaluated 40 patients with a diagnosis of CD with both CCE and ileocolonoscopy. Using the Crohn's Disease Endoscopic Index of Severity, each patient was scored for active colitis with both tools. The investigators reported significant agreement between the 2 methods with an intraclass correlation coefficient (ICC) of 0.65 (95% confidence interval [CI] 0.43–0.80). The agreement between the 2 methods was more significant in the terminal ileum, where the ICC reached 0.73 (95% CI 0.54–0.85). In the colon, there was less agreement, with a tendency for CCE to underestimate severity. Overall, the CCE was tolerated better by patients compared with ileocolonoscopy.[63]

The more recent development of PCE has been the next logical step for CE in patients with CD. Unlike the CCE, the PCE is designed to evaluate both the small bowel and colon. A recent feasibility study documented performance of PCE that exceeded ileocolonoscopy with statistical significance in 66 patients who underwent both modalities. The diagnostic yield per patient for PCE was higher than that of ileocolonoscopy at rates of 83.3% and 69.7%, respectively.[64] Preliminary data from a study comparing PCE with MRE and ileocolonoscopy in pediatric patients with CD suggests that it may be highly sensitive for both small bowel and colonic mucosal lesions, and is more tolerable for patients than both MRE and ileocolonoscopy.[65] Many questions remain to be answered regarding both the CCE and the PCE before they find their way into routine practice in the management of CD.

CAPSULE RETENTION

In general, CE is a very low-risk procedure with one major exception: retention of the video capsule. The risk of capsule retention in the general population is probably very low, and estimates of its incidence range from 1.0% to 2.5%.[50,66–68] Predictably, in the evaluation of patients with CD this rate is higher, owing to the higher incidence of gastrointestinal strictures in this population.[69] The cited risk of retention in suspected CD is not much higher than in the general population, occurring at a rate of 2.6%.[70] In patients with established CD, the rate is unsurprisingly higher. As we have discussed, this patient population is the one in which CE may be most useful in guiding management. It is therefore important that patients with established CE be pre-screened for potential capsule retention before undergoing CE. A capsule retention rate as high as 13% in patients with established CD has been recorded in older literature.[70] Current practice indicates that patients with suspected CD at risk for capsule retention and patients with established CD undergo a pre-CE screening with either a patency capsule or cross-sectional imaging. One documented drawback to the use of patency capsule is its substantial false positive rate.[71,72] One method for improving on this measure is the use of radiologic imaging to confirm the location of the capsule as either in the small bowel, or more safely located in the colon. The use of low dose or "spot" CT has demonstrated utility in this area. In one retrospective study, 16 (66%) of 24 patients with a positive patency capsule who underwent spot CT subsequently underwent CE with no instance of retained capsule.[73] More recent meta-analysis probably reflects current pre-CE screening practices in citing retention rates of 2.45% in suspected CD and 4.63% in established CD. The same study further clarified that the risk of retention is substantially reduced in those patients with established CD who were screened for retention before CE. The rate of retention for patients who had undergone small bowel cross-sectional imaging before CE was 2.32%, and for those who had a patency capsule the rate of retention was 2.88%.[74] For all patients with established CD, the risk of capsule retention should be reviewed and informed consent should be obtained before CE, even when cross-sectional imaging studies are normal.[11,75,76]

The first-line management of the retained capsule should be medical, and surgery should be avoided if at all possible. A conservative, observational approach is the first treatment for the retained capsule, as many will pass spontaneously.[77] When necessary, medical therapy in the form of steroids and biologic agents has proven helpful, particularly in the patient with IBD.[67,77,78] Retrieval of the capsule, either endoscopically or surgically, should be reserved for those patients in whom observation and medical therapy have failed.[79]

PREPARATION OF THE BOWEL

Evidence is substantial that the use of a bowel preparation before CE improves visualization and diagnostic yield. One study that reviewed 15 randomized controlled trials documented that, when compared with no preparation, bowel preparation with polyethylene glycol (PEG) significantly improved the odds of visualization of the bowel (odds ratio [OR] 3.13; 95% CI 1.70–5.75; $P = .002$) and improved the diagnostic yield (46.4% with PEG vs 36.2% with no preparation, OR 1.68; 95% CI 1.16–2.42; $P = .006$). The same review cited an improved diagnostic yield with use of sodium phosphate as preparation (OR 1.77; 95% CI 1.18–2.64; $P = .005$).[80] Based on these data, current guidelines recommend that all patients undergoing CE take a bowel preparation before their examination.[81] Yet the use of preparations in small bowel CE remains controversial. A meta-analysis of 40 studies analyzed bowel preparations in CE of the small bowel and found that they did not significantly improve diagnostic yield (OR 1.10; 95% CI 0.85–1.44) and only modestly improved visualization (OR 1.60; 95% CI 1.08–2.06).[82]

In the cases of CCE and PCE, appropriate visualization of the colonic mucosa can be more challenging. One obvious limitation of CE in the colon relative to traditional endoscopic technique is the inability to actively wash and suction debris, necessitating an adequate bowel preparation. In addition, the capsule itself has limited battery life and adjunctive therapies must be used to assist in propelling the capsule through the colon.[83,84] For these reasons, the current practice of bowel preparation in these patients is more aggressive compared with that used in patients undergoing standard colonoscopy. The most frequently used regimens use split dosing of PEG combined with sodium phosphate (NaP) and a prokinetic agent in the form of boosters often followed by a bisacodyl suppository.[83–88]

SUMMARY

The role of CE in IBD continues to evolve with advancing technology. CE in its current form provides consistent, high-quality visual images of the small bowel mucosa. It is a highly sensitive tool for mucosal disruptions in the small bowel, and as such is a powerful negative predictive tool. Although it is low in specificity, this value can be improved with biomarkers such as fecal calprotectin. CE is tolerated well by patients, and is a low-risk procedure overall. The important complication of the procedure is capsule retention, which is dependent on the indication for the examination. The overall retention rate is still low, and screening for retention should involve a thorough history taking regarding previous surgeries, chronic NSAID usage, and previous or current obstructions. The use of cross-sectional imaging of the abdomen and/or the administration of a patency capsule before CE can reduce the rate of retention in patients with risk factors.

In the current environment, CE probably finds its greatest utility in the surveillance of patients with CD. The goal of mucosal healing in IBD is an endpoint of disease management that has superseded that of clinical improvement. To that end, endoscopic surveillance is a pillar of therapy, and CE is a minimally invasive device designed for that objective. There remains a need for a validated scoring mechanism that would allow for standardized evaluation.

Outside of established CD, there are still areas in which CE may find itself useful. Patients with IBDU or those in whom IBD is highly suspected despite negative ileocolonoscopy can potentially benefit from a CE examination. In addition, there is an increasing role for CE in UC. Small bowel lesions can be seen in patients with UC, which can correlate with disease activity in the colon, or can be helpful in the diagnosis and management of patients with UC after colectomy. Moreover, the development and refinement of the CCE and PCE may help us to monitor UC in the colon, while at the same time identifying small bowel lesions. There remains much research and improvement to be made in this area before CE becomes standard practice in the management of UC.

CLINICS CARE POINTS

- CE is useful in diagnosis of small bowel CD in patients with negative ileocolonoscopy.
- CE is useful in evaluation of patients with established CD to evaluate small bowel disease extent and activity.
- CE may be useful in diagnosis of CD in patients with IBDU.
- CE may be useful to evaluate for postoperative recurrence of CD in patients with a negative ileocolonoscopy.
- In the absence of obstructive symptoms and other risk factors, CE carries a low risk of retention in patients with suspected CD.
- CE has a high risk of retention in established CD even in the absence of obstructive symptoms.
- The performance of patency capsule or dedicated small bowel cross-sectional imaging significantly reduces risk of capsule retention.

DISCLOSURE

J.D. McCain: no disclosures. S.F. Pasha: Medtronic: research and consulting; Olympus: consulting. J.A. Leighton: Olympus: consulting.

SUPPLEMENTARY DATA

Supplementary data related to this article can be found online at https://doi.org/10.1016/j.giec.2020.12.004.

REFERENCES

1. Valle J, Alcántara M, Pérez-Grueso MJ, et al. Clinical features of patients with negative results from traditional diagnostic work-up and Crohn's disease findings from capsule endoscopy. J Clin Gastroenterol 2006;40(8):692–6.
2. Vavricka SR, Spigaglia SM, Rogler G, et al. Systematic evaluation of risk factors for diagnostic delay in inflammatory bowel disease. Inflamm Bowel Dis 2012; 18(3):496–505.
3. Triester SL, Leighton JA, Leontiadis GI, et al. A meta-analysis of the yield of capsule endoscopy compared to other diagnostic modalities in patients with non-stricturing small bowel Crohn's disease. Am J Gastroenterol 2006;101(5): 954–64.
4. Dionisio PM, Gurudu SR, Leighton JA, et al. Capsule endoscopy has a significantly higher diagnostic yield in patients with suspected and established small-bowel Crohn's disease: a meta-analysis. Am J Gastroenterol 2010;105(6): 1240–8 [quiz 9].
5. Herrerías JM, Caunedo A, Rodríguez-Téllez M, et al. Capsule endoscopy in patients with suspected Crohn's disease and negative endoscopy. Endoscopy 2003;35(7):564–8.
6. Fireman Z, Mahajna E, Broide E, et al. Diagnosing small bowel Crohn's disease with wireless capsule endoscopy. Gut 2003;52(3):390–2.
7. Mow WS, Lo SK, Targan SR, et al. Initial experience with wireless capsule enteroscopy in the diagnosis and management of inflammatory bowel disease. Clin Gastroenterol Hepatol 2004;2(1):31–40.
8. Marmo R, Rotondano G, Piscopo R, et al. Capsule endoscopy versus enteroclysis in the detection of small-bowel involvement in Crohn's disease: a prospective trial. Clin Gastroenterol Hepatol 2005;3(8):772–6.
9. Khater NH, Fahmy HS, Ali HI. Value of MR enterography in assessment of Crohn's disease: correlation with capsule endoscopy and colonoscopy. The Egyptian Journal of Radiology and Nuclear Medicine 2017;48(1):51–60.
10. González-Suárez B, Rodriguez S, Ricart E, et al. Comparison of capsule endoscopy and magnetic resonance enterography for the assessment of small bowel lesions in crohn's disease. Inflamm Bowel Dis 2018;24(4):775–80.
11. Solem CA, Loftus EV Jr, Fletcher JG, et al. Small-bowel imaging in Crohn's disease: a prospective, blinded, 4-way comparison trial. Gastrointest Endosc 2008;68(2):255–66.
12. Jensen MD, Nathan T, Rafaelsen SR, et al. Diagnostic accuracy of capsule endoscopy for small bowel Crohn's disease is superior to that of MR enterography or CT enterography. Clin Gastroenterol Hepatol 2011;9(2):124–9.
13. Girelli CM, Porta P, Malacrida V, et al. Clinical outcome of patients examined by capsule endoscopy for suspected small bowel Crohn's disease. Dig Liver Dis 2007;39(2):148–54.
14. Koulaouzidis A, Douglas S, Rogers MA, et al. Fecal calprotectin: a selection tool for small bowel capsule endoscopy in suspected IBD with prior negative bidirectional endoscopy. Scand J Gastroenterol 2011;46(5):561–6.

15. Höög CM, Bark L, Broström O, et al. Capsule endoscopic findings correlate with fecal calprotectin and C-reactive protein in patients with suspected small-bowel Crohn's disease. Scand J Gastroenterol 2014;49(9):1084–90.
16. Monteiro S, Barbosa M, Cúrdia Gonçalves T, et al. Fecal calprotectin as a selection tool for small bowel capsule endoscopy in suspected crohn's disease. Inflamm Bowel Dis 2018;24(9):2033–8.
17. Hall B, Holleran G, Costigan D, et al. Capsule endoscopy: high negative predictive value in the long term despite a low diagnostic yield in patients with suspected Crohn's disease. United Eur Gastroenterol J 2013;1(6):461–6.
18. Goldstein JL, Eisen GM, Lewis B, et al. Video capsule endoscopy to prospectively assess small bowel injury with celecoxib, naproxen plus omeprazole, and placebo. Clin Gastroenterol Hepatol 2005;3(2):133–41.
19. Dilauro S, Crum-Cianflone NF. Ileitis: when it is not Crohn's disease. Curr Gastroenterol Rep 2010;12(4):249–58.
20. Capurso G, Lahner E, Pallotta N, et al. Iron deficiency anaemia caused by nonspecific (idiopathic) small bowel ulceration: an uncommon presentation of an uncommon disease. Can J Gastroenterol 2002;16:451641.
21. Bouguen G, Levesque BG, Feagan BG, et al. Treat to target: a proposed new paradigm for the management of Crohn's disease. Clin Gastroenterol Hepatol 2015;13(6):1042–50.e2.
22. Gralnek IM, Defranchis R, Seidman E, et al. Development of a capsule endoscopy scoring index for small bowel mucosal inflammatory change. Aliment Pharmacol Ther 2008;27(2):146–54.
23. Gal E, Geller A, Fraser G, et al. Assessment and validation of the new capsule endoscopy Crohn's disease activity index (CECDAI). Dig Dis Sci 2008;53(7):1933–7.
24. Rosa B, Pinho R, de Ferro SM, et al. Endoscopic scores for evaluation of crohn's disease activity at small bowel capsule endoscopy: general principles and current applications. GE Port J Gastroenterol 2016;23(1):36–41.
25. Omori T, Kambayashi H, Murasugi S, et al. Comparison of lewis score and capsule endoscopy crohn's disease activity index in patients with Crohn's disease. Dig Dis Sci 2020;65(4):1180–8.
26. Yablecovitch D, Lahat A, Neuman S, et al. The Lewis score or the capsule endoscopy Crohn's disease activity index: which one is better for the assessment of small bowel inflammation in established Crohn's disease? Ther Adv Gastroenterol 2018;11. 1756283X17747780-1756283X.
27. Efthymiou A, Viazis N, Mantzaris G, et al. Does clinical response correlate with mucosal healing in patients with Crohn's disease of the small bowel? A prospective, case-series study using wireless capsule endoscopy. Inflamm Bowel Dis 2008;14(11):1542–7.
28. Niv Y. Diagnostic value of capsule endoscopy during relapse in co-morbid irritable bowel syndrome and Crohn's disease. Eur J Gastroenterol Hepatol 2004;16(10):1073–4.
29. Costamagna G, Shah SK, Riccioni ME, et al. A prospective trial comparing small bowel radiographs and video capsule endoscopy for suspected small bowel disease. Gastroenterology 2002;123(4):999–1005.
30. Voderholzer WA, Beinhoelzl J, Rogalla P, et al. Small bowel involvement in Crohn's disease: a prospective comparison of wireless capsule endoscopy and computed tomography enteroclysis. Gut 2005;54(3):369–73.

31. Albert JG, Martiny F, Krummenerl A, et al. Diagnosis of small bowel Crohn's disease: a prospective comparison of capsule endoscopy with magnetic resonance imaging and fluoroscopic enteroclysis. Gut 2005;54(12):1721–7.

32. Flamant M, Trang C, Maillard O, et al. The prevalence and outcome of jejunal lesions visualized by small bowel capsule endoscopy in Crohn's disease. Inflamm Bowel Dis 2013;19(7):1390–6.

33. Doherty GA, Moss AC, Cheifetz AS. Capsule endoscopy for small-bowel evaluation in Crohn's disease. Gastrointest Endosc 2011;74(1):167–75.

34. Bourreille A, Jarry M, D'Halluin PN, et al. Wireless capsule endoscopy versus ileocolonoscopy for the diagnosis of postoperative recurrence of Crohn's disease: a prospective study. Gut 2006;55(7):978–83.

35. Pons Beltrán V, Nos P, Bastida G, et al. Evaluation of postsurgical recurrence in Crohn's disease: a new indication for capsule endoscopy? Gastrointest Endosc 2007;66(3):533–40.

36. Lo S, Zaidel O, Tabibzadeh S, et al. Utility of wireless capsule enteroscopy (WCE) and IBD serology in reclassifying indeterminate colitis (IC). Gastroenterology 2003;124.

37. Ge Z-Z, Hu Y-B, Xiao S-D. Capsule endoscopy in diagnosis of small bowel Crohn's disease. World J Gastroenterol 2004;10(9):1349–52.

38. Maunoury V, Savoye G, Bourreille A, et al. Value of wireless capsule endoscopy in patients with indeterminate colitis (inflammatory bowel disease type unclassified). Inflamm Bowel Dis 2007;13(2):152–5.

39. Mehdizadeh S, Chen G, Enayati PJ, et al. Diagnostic yield of capsule endoscopy in ulcerative colitis and inflammatory bowel disease of unclassified type (IBDU). Endoscopy 2008;40(1):30–5.

40. Lopes S, Figueiredo P, Portela F, et al. Capsule endoscopy in inflammatory bowel disease type unclassified and indeterminate colitis serologically negative. Inflamm Bowel Dis 2010;16(10):1663–8.

41. Di Nardo G, Oliva S, Ferrari F, et al. Usefulness of wireless capsule endoscopy in paediatric inflammatory bowel disease. Dig Liver Dis 2011;43(3):220–4.

42. Frøslie KF, Jahnsen J, Moum BA, et al. Mucosal healing in inflammatory bowel disease: results from a Norwegian population-based cohort. Gastroenterology 2007;133(2):412–22.

43. Melmed GY, Dubinsky MC, Rubin DT, et al. Utility of video capsule endoscopy for longitudinal monitoring of Crohn's disease activity in the small bowel: a prospective study. Gastrointest Endosc 2018;88(6):947–55.e2.

44. Deabes A, Gavin M. Obscure occult GI bleeding: an iatrogenic tale? Dig Dis Sci 2016;61(1):42–5.

45. Tachecí I, Bradna P, Douda T, et al. NSAID-induced enteropathy in rheumatoid arthritis patients with chronic occult gastrointestinal bleeding: a prospective capsule endoscopy study. Gastroenterol Res Pract 2013;2013:268382.

46. Graham DY, Opekun AR, Willingham FF, et al. Visible small-intestinal mucosal injury in chronic NSAID users. Clin Gastroenterol Hepatol 2005;3(1):55–9.

47. Courtenay L, Kwok A, Keshava A. Gastrointestinal: diaphragm disease: emerging cause of gastrointestinal obstruction and bleeding. J Gastroenterol Hepatol 2014; 29(2):230.

48. Frye JM, Hansel SL, Dolan SG, et al. NSAID enteropathy: appearance at CT and MR enterography in the age of multi-modality imaging and treatment. Abdom Imaging 2015;40(5):1011–25.

49. Lim YJ, Yang C-H. Non-steroidal anti-inflammatory drug-induced enteropathy. Clin Endosc 2012;45(2):138–44.

50. Li F, Gurudu SR, De Petris G, et al. Retention of the capsule endoscope: a single-center experience of 1000 capsule endoscopy procedures. Gastrointest Endosc 2008;68(1):174–80.
51. Schembri J, Azzopardi M, Ellul P. Small bowel radiation enteritis diagnosed by capsule endoscopy. BMJ Case Rep 2014;2014. bcr2013202552.
52. Lee DW, Poon AO, Chan AC. Diagnosis of small bowel radiation enteritis by capsule endoscopy. Hong Kong Med J 2004;10(6):419–21.
53. Nakamura M, Hirooka Y, Watanabe O, et al. Three cases with active bleeding from radiation enteritis that were diagnosed with video capsule endoscopy without retention. Nagoya J Med Sci 2014;76(3–4):369–74.
54. Kim HM, Kim YJ, Kim HJ, et al. A pilot study of capsule endoscopy for the diagnosis of radiation enteritis. Hepatogastroenterology 2011;58(106):459–64.
55. Sousa M, Pinho R, Proença L. Capsule endoscopy in the diagnosis of eosinophilic enteritis. GE Port J Gastroenterol 2019;26(5):381–2.
56. Herrera Quiñones G, Scharrer SI, Jiménez Rodríguez AR, et al. Diagnosis of eosinophilic enteritis with video capsule endoscopy and double balloon enteroscopy with favorable response to corticosteroids. ACG case Rep J 2019;6(7): e00127-e.
57. Okuda K, Daimon Y, Iwase T, et al. Novel findings of capsule endoscopy and double-balloon enteroscopy in a case of eosinophilic gastroenteritis. Clin J Gastroenterol 2013;6(1):16–9.
58. Akram S, Murray JA, Pardi DS, et al. Adult autoimmune enteropathy: Mayo Clinic Rochester experience. Clin Gastroenterol Hepatol 2007;5(11):1282–90.
59. Gram-Kampmann E-M, Lillevang ST, Detlefsen S, et al. Wireless capsule endoscopy as a tool in diagnosing autoimmune enteropathy. BMJ Case Rep 2015;2015. bcr2014207931.
60. Oliva S, Di Nardo G, Hassan C, et al. Second-generation colon capsule endoscopy vs. colonoscopy in pediatric ulcerative colitis: a pilot study. Endoscopy 2014;46(06):485–92.
61. Sung J, Ho KY, Chiu HM, et al. The use of Pillcam Colon in assessing mucosal inflammation in ulcerative colitis: a multicenter study. Endoscopy 2012;44(8): 754–8.
62. Shi HY, Chan FKL, Higashimori A, et al. A prospective study on second-generation colon capsule endoscopy to detect mucosal lesions and disease activity in ulcerative colitis (with video). Gastrointest Endosc 2017;86(6): 1139–46.e6.
63. D'Haens G, Löwenberg M, Samaan MA, et al. Safety and feasibility of using the second-generation Pillcam colon capsule to assess active colonic Crohn's disease. Clin Gastroenterol Hepatol 2015;13(8):1480–6.e3.
64. Leighton JA, Helper DJ, Gralnek IM, et al. Comparing diagnostic yield of a novel pan-enteric video capsule endoscope with ileocolonoscopy in patients with active Crohn's disease: a feasibility study. Gastrointest Endosc 2017;85(1): 196–205.e1.
65. Oliva S, Cucchiara S, Aloi M, et al. 288 Pan-enteric capsule endoscopy in pediatric Crohn's disease – the ped-pan study: preliminary results of a multicenter trial. Gastrointest Endosc 2019;89(6). AB66-AB7.
66. Baichi MM, Arifuddin RM, Mantry PS. What we have learned from 5 cases of permanent capsule retention. Gastrointest Endosc 2006;64(2):283–7.
67. Cheon JH, Kim YS, Lee IS, et al. Can we predict spontaneous capsule passage after retention? A nationwide study to evaluate the incidence and clinical outcomes of capsule retention. Endoscopy 2007;39(12):1046–52.

68. Karagiannis S, Faiss S, Mavrogiannis C. Capsule retention: a feared complication of wireless capsule endoscopy. Scand J Gastroenterol 2009;44(10):1158–65.

69. Liao Z, Gao R, Xu C, et al. Indications and detection, completion, and retention rates of small-bowel capsule endoscopy: a systematic review. Gastrointest Endosc 2010;71(2):280–6.

70. Cheifetz AS, Kornbluth AA, Legnani P, et al. The risk of retention of the capsule endoscope in patients with known or suspected Crohn's disease. Am J Gastroenterol 2006;101(10):2218–22.

71. Yadav A, Heigh RI, Hara AK, et al. Performance of the patency capsule compared with nonenteroclysis radiologic examinations in patients with known or suspected intestinal strictures. Gastrointest Endosc 2011;74(4):834–9.

72. Sawada T, Nakamura M, Watanabe O, et al. Clinical factors related to false-positive rates of patency capsule examination. Ther Adv Gastroenterol 2017; 10(8):589–98.

73. Yadav A, Hara A, Russel H, et al. Utility of low radiation dose spot CT as a screening test to localize retained patency capsules and reduce false-positive results: 307. Am J Gastroenterol 2012;107:S131.

74. Pasha SF, Pennazio M, Rondonotti E, et al. Capsule retention in Crohn's disease: a meta-analysis. Inflamm Bowel Dis 2020;26(1):33–42.

75. Figueiredo P, Almeida N, Lopes S, et al. Small-bowel capsule endoscopy in patients with suspected Crohn's disease-diagnostic value and complications. Diagn Ther Endosc 2010;2010:101284.

76. Hara AK, Leighton JA, Heigh RI, et al. Crohn disease of the small bowel: preliminary comparison among CT enterography, capsule endoscopy, small-bowel follow-through, and ileoscopy. Radiology 2006;238(1):128–34.

77. Fernández-Urién I, Carretero C, González B, et al. Incidence, clinical outcomes, and therapeutic approaches of capsule endoscopy-related adverse events in a large study population. Rev Esp Enferm Dig 2015;107(12):745–52.

78. Vanfleteren L, van der Schaar P, Goedhard J. Ileus related to wireless capsule retention in suspected Crohn's disease: emergency surgery obviated by early pharmacological treatment. Endoscopy 2009;41(S 02):E134–5.

79. Rondonotti E. Capsule retention: prevention, diagnosis and management. Ann transl Med 2017;5(9):198.

80. Kotwal VS, Attar BM, Gupta S, et al. Should bowel preparation, antifoaming agents, or prokinetics be used before video capsule endoscopy? A systematic review and meta-analysis. Eur J Gastroenterol Hepatol 2014;26(2):137–45.

81. Enns RA, Hookey L, Armstrong D, et al. Clinical practice guidelines for the use of video capsule endoscopy. Gastroenterology 2017;152(3):497–514.

82. Yung DE, Rondonotti E, Sykes C, et al. Systematic review and meta-analysis: is bowel preparation still necessary in small bowel capsule endoscopy? Expert Rev Gastroenterol Hepatol 2017;11(10):979–93.

83. Spada C, Riccioni ME, Hassan C, et al. PillCam colon capsule endoscopy: a prospective, randomized trial comparing two regimens of preparation. J Clin Gastroenterol 2011;45(2):119–24.

84. Singhal S, Nigar S, Paleti V, et al. Bowel preparation regimens for colon capsule endoscopy: a review. Ther Adv Gastroenterol 2013;7(3):115–22.

85. Eliakim R, Yassin K, Niv Y, et al. Prospective multicenter performance evaluation of the second-generation colon capsule compared with colonoscopy. Endoscopy 2009;41(12):1026–31.

86. Van Gossum A, Munoz-Navas M, Fernandez-Urien I, et al. Capsule endoscopy versus colonoscopy for the detection of polyps and cancer. N Engl J Med 2009;361(3):264–70.
87. Usui S, Hosoe N, Matsuoka K, et al. Modified bowel preparation regimen for use in second-generation colon capsule endoscopy in patients with ulcerative colitis. Dig Endosc 2014;26(5):665–72.
88. Spada C, Hassan C, Ingrosso M, et al. A new regimen of bowel preparation for PillCam colon capsule endoscopy: a pilot study. Dig Liver Dis 2011;43(4):300–4.

The Role of Video Capsule Endoscopy in Liver Disease

Alexander Ross Robertson, MBChB, MRCP, AFHEA[a],
Anastasios Koulaouzidis, MD, MD(Res), PhD, FEBG[b], Emanuele Rondonotti, MD, PhD[c],
Mauro Bruno, MD[d], Marco Pennazio, MD[d],*

KEYWORDS

- Capsule endoscopy • Cirrhosis • Portal hypertension • Varices • Enteropathy
- Panenteric • Surveillance

KEY POINTS

- Endoscopy has a wide range of diagnostic and therapeutic roles in patients with liver disease.
- Capsule endoscopy is recognized as a viable alternative in patients unable or unwilling to undergo upper gastrointestinal endoscopy.
- Anemia is common in chronic and advanced liver disease, observed in approximately 75% of cases.
- Alterations in capsule design is leading to ever-improving detection of panenteric complications of portal hypertension.

 Video content accompanies this article at http://www.giendo.theclinics.com.

BACKGROUND

Endoscopy has a wide range of diagnostic and therapeutic roles in patients with liver disease. Variceal bleeding is one of the most common and severe complications of liver cirrhosis. Even with the current best medical care, mortality from variceal bleeding remains at approximately 20%.[1] Moreover, variceal bleeding often leads to deterioration in liver function and is a common trigger for other complications of cirrhosis, such as bacterial infection or hepatorenal syndrome. Varices are present in 30% to 40% of

[a] Department of Gastroenterology, Western General Hospital, Crewe Road South, Edinburgh EH4 2XU, Scotland; [b] Pomeranian Medical University, Department of Social Medicine & Public Health, Faculty of Health Sciences, Rybacka 1, Szczecin, West Pomeranian Voivodeship, Poland; [c] Gastroenterology Unit, Valduce Hospital, Dante Alighieri Street, 11, Como 22100, Italy; [d] University Division of Gastroenterology, City of Health and Science University Hospital, Via Cavour 31, 10123 Turin, Italy
* Corresponding author.
E-mail address: pennazio.marco@gmail.com
Twitter: @alexoscopy (A.R.R.)

Gastrointest Endoscopy Clin N Am 31 (2021) 363–376
https://doi.org/10.1016/j.giec.2020.12.007
1052-5157/21/© 2020 Elsevier Inc. All rights reserved.

patients with compensated cirrhosis and 60% of those who present with ascites. The annual incidence of new varices in those with cirrhosis who present initially without is approximately 5% to 10%.[2] At present, upper gastrointestinal (GI) endoscopy represents the gold standard for the screening, treatment, and surveillance of esophageal varices. Endoscopy, however, is still perceived by patients as an invasive and unpleasant examination, and so in the past few years, several attempts have been made to better stratify the risk of developing portal hypertension and to identify those who can safely avoid screening and surveillance endoscopy.[3] Where screening/surveillance of esophageal varices is indicated, capsule endoscopy might represent a less invasive alternative to upper GI endoscopy.

In patients with portal hypertension due to liver cirrhosis, anemia is much more frequently observed than in the general population. In these patients, conventional endoscopy (ie, upper and lower GI endoscopy) often represents the first diagnostic step, but is often suboptimal for identifying the source of blood loss and evaluation of the small bowel (SB) is required. In addition, SB abnormalities are increasingly common with advancing liver disease and seen in 87% of video capsule endoscopy (VCE) in the lead up to liver transplantation[4] and in almost all cirrhotic patients in studies using the newest technologies.[5] Despite this, portal hypertension–related SB disease has traditionally been underrecognized, largely because of its inaccessibility. Portal hypertension–related abnormalities develop with clinically significant portal hypertension, as the hepatic venous pressure gradient raises more than 10 mm Hg.[6] The most common portal hypertension findings in the SB are villous edema, red spots, angioectasia, erosions, and varices.[7–9] Nowadays these findings are easily recognized and evaluated by means of VCE.

Patients with liver cirrhosis are often frail and lacking physiologic reserve, are at a higher risk for general anesthetic, and have been seen to have a 4 to 5 times higher mortality in emergency surgery.[10] As such, minimally invasive technologies are highly appealing. VCE is safe and well tolerated in those with advanced liver disease, both adults and children, without the need for sedation.[11,12] Last but not least, those with liver disease are not considered to be at a higher risk of capsule retention and VCE has a completion rate comparable to the general population.[4,13] Therefore, it can be used to establish a diagnosis and guide the need for more invasive management or therapy.

CAPSULE ENDOSCOPY IN DIAGNOSIS AND SURVEILLANCE OF PORTAL HYPERTENSION

Many patients struggle to tolerate upper GI endoscopy, and this results in suboptimal visualization and a poorer-quality study. Many will decline either initial or repeat examination based on their perception of the procedure or previous discomfort, and surveillance programs often necessitate repeated procedures over many years. VCE often represents an acceptable and well-tolerated alternative to patients of all ages[12,14] (**Fig. 1**, Video 1).

For this purpose, a dedicated capsule (PillCam ESO; Given Imaging, Yokneam, Israel), specifically designed for the study of the esophagus, has been released. This capsule is 11 × 26 mm in size and has 2 cameras that are able to acquire images from both ends of the device during its passage through the esophagus. These are recorded at a rate of 7 frames per second per camera (or at 9 frames per second per camera: PillCam Eso2; Given Imaging), images at this rate for 20 minutes. To slow down the esophageal transit and to decrease the presence of bubbles and/or saliva, a specific ingestion protocol has been designed. This protocol requires placing

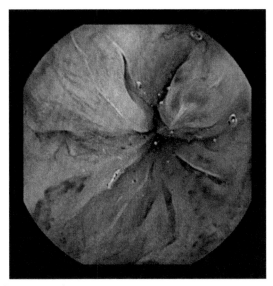

Fig. 1. Esophageal varices with VCE.

the patient on a bed with the top tilted at different inclinations following a strict time schedule. The original ingestion protocol worked well in the initial studies, but gave mixed results on routine application. This was possibly related to deviation from the protocol, given the inconvenience of ingesting the capsule in a supine position. Therefore, a simplified ingestion procedure was devised in which the patient lies on a right lateral decubitus position throughout the procedure and sips 10 mL of water every 30 seconds with a straw.[15]

To increase the capability of the capsule in identifying findings in the esophagus, investigators have suggested attaching a soft string to an SB capsule. This technique allows the capsule to be moved up and down the esophagus by gently moving the string, thus allowing a clear view of the distal esophagus. In addition, because of its 8 hours of battery life, the string capsule can be retrieved via the patient's mouth, and after cleaning and disinfection, stored, and re-used to examine several patients. The string capsule has mostly been used for patients with signs of gastroesophageal reflux disease, dysphagia, or Barrett's esophagus.[16,17] To the best of our knowledge, there is only 1 full article[18] that describes this technique for patients with esophageal varices. Although the performance of the string capsule in recognizing the presence of varices was impressive (96% sensitivity, 100% specificity, positive and negative predictive values 100% and 83%, respectively) in this study, the limited sample size made it difficult to reach any firm conclusion.

Recently, an updated system (PillCam UGI; Medtronic, Dublin, Ireland) with a longer battery life and variable frame rate (up to 35 frames per second) has been marketed. The use of magnetically steerable capsules[15] as well as a combination of the latter with a detachable string, has also been proposed.[19,20] Nevertheless, the trials with these new capsules are mostly focused on technical issues and most clinical studies published so far (and summarized in the next few paragraphs) have been performed with the first and the second generation of esophageal capsule.

Most studies focused on esophageal varices involve a relatively small population, are performed in tertiary referral centers, and show a wide variability, both in terms of sensitivity and specificity. Therefore, in an effort to evaluate the performance of esophageal capsule endoscopy in larger studies, a meta-analysis was released in 2017 by McCarty and colleagues.[11] This reported a diagnostic accuracy of 90% for VCE in diagnosing esophageal varices with a sensitivity of 83% and specificity of 85%. Although the accuracy was 92% for clinically significant (medium-large varices that required a change to management), this article concluded that capsule endoscopy was not currently sufficient to replace gastroscopy[11] (see **Table 1**). Importantly, this meta-analysis reported only 2 adverse events, which both related to capsule retention in unsuspected esophageal strictures.

A Cochrane review found similar results, including 6 studies into the detection of large, clinically significant varices. With VCE, the pooled sensitivity was 73.7% and specificity 90.5% (see **Table 2**). They did, however, also recognize the very low rates of complications or adverse events and that participants reported this to be well tolerated.[21] As such, VCE is recognized as a suboptimal but safe and better tolerated investigation for esophageal varices. It will likely continue to have a role in those who are unwilling or unable to tolerate a conventional endoscopy, which remains the gold standard.

Further to this, surveillance of children with portal hypertension is associated with difficulties. Although VCE is a relatively safe option for surveillance,[12] this does remain controvertial.[22] In children, primary prophylaxis for variceal bleeding is safe and effective, once high-risk features have been identified.[23] This is important, as following a first spontaneous variceal bleed as many as 19% of children develop life-threatening complications[23] and VCE in this setting is seen to change management.[22,24]

Magnetically assisted capsule endoscopy (MACE) technology using a MiroCam Navi (Intromedic Ltd, Seoul, Korea) capsule successfully allows a device to be held in the esophagus. Despite this, the sensitivity was only 73.3% (11 of 15) and specificity 100% in identifying esophageal varices.[25]

VCE performs poorly in identifying *gastric varices*, recognizing 0% in a series of 13 reported by Krok and colleagues.[26] This article showed a similar success in detecting esophageal varices to the meta-analyses mentioned previously, whereas the poor diagnostic performance in detecting gastric varices was attributed to the lack of insufflations and to the passive uncontrolled capsule movements in a wide lumen organ, see **Fig. 2**. MACE, however, seems to offer a solution. Using an external magnetic control system to alter the view of the capsule, it is possible to improve visualization of the fundus and assess for varices. However, the lack of adequate insufflation still remains a relevant issue, even with magnetically controlled capsules, and views of the fundus remain poor compared with the rest of the gastric mucosa. Although this process has been seen, in the framework of preliminary feasibility study, to detect gastric varices in 2 patients who had refused conventional gastroscopic, larger studies are required.[27]

Table 1
Pooled accuracy in diagnosing esophageal varices with VCE

Varices	Diagnostic Accuracy	Sensitivity	Specificity
All esophageal varices	90% (95% CI 0.88–0.93)	83% (95% CI 0.76–0.89)	85% (95% CI 0.75–0.91)
Medium to large varices	92% (95% CI 0.90–0.94)	72% (95% CI 0.54–0.85)	91% (95% CI 0.86–0.94)

Abbreviations: CI, confidence interval; VCE, video capsule endoscopy.
From McCarty TR, Afinogenova Y, Njei B. Use of wireless capsule endoscopy for the diagnosis and grading of esophageal varices in patients with portal hypertension: A systematic review and meta-analysis. *J Clin Gastroenterol.* 2017; with permission.

Table 2
Pooled accuracy in diagnosing esophageal varices with VCE

Varices	Sensitivity, %	Specificity, %
All esophageal varices	84.8 (95 CI 77.3–90.2)	84.3 (95 CI 73.1–91.4)
Large varices	73.7 (95 CI 52.4–87.7)	90.5 (95 CI 84.1–94.4)

Abbreviations: CI, confidence interval; VCE, video capsule endoscopy.
From Colli A, Gana JC, Turner D, et al. Capsule endoscopy for the diagnosis of oesophageal varices in people with chronic liver disease or portal vein thrombosis. *Cochrane Database Syst Rev.* 2014; with permission.

Portal hypertensive gastropathy (PHG) is seen in 20% to 80% of those with cirrhosis, with increasing rates in those having previously undergone variceal ligation and more advanced liver disease[28] (see **Fig. 3**). There is increased mucosal blood flow with vascular dilatation within the mucosa/submucosa, and those with PHG have between an 8% and 25% annual risk of bleeding, depending on the severity of the PHG.[29] In studies, when adequate views are obtained, VCE shows good specificity and sensitivity for PHG (95.1% for both), although significant numbers of procedures did not give adequate views of the gastric mucosa, and so often no judgment could be given.[26]

Gastric antral vascular ectasia (GAVE), commonly referred to as "watermelon stomach," can appear very similar to PHG and accounts for approximately 5% of nonvariceal upper GI bleeding (see **Fig. 4**). GAVE is formed of tortuous ectatic vessels in the antral folds and does not necessarily coincide with liver disease, but rather can be seen in a variety of conditions, including those of the kidneys or connective tissue. When associated with liver disease, it seems to resolve after liver transplantation.[30]

GAVE is well observed on VCE, possibly due to close view of the antral mucosa, as the capsule often remains in this position for extended periods before passing through the pylorus. In addition, the lack of air insufflation allows improved visualization of the

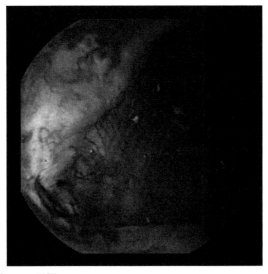

Fig. 2. Gastric varices on VCE.

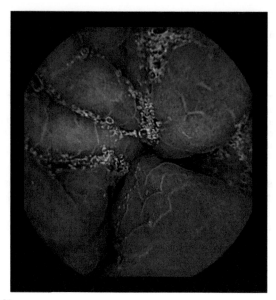

Fig. 3. PHG on VCE.

prominent vascularity when compared with conventional esophago-gastro duodeno-scopy (EGD).[31]

Gastric and duodenal portal hypertensive polyposis are potential causes of bleeding. Portal hypertensive polyps commonly recur after resection but do not seem to undergo malignant transformation when followed up. One study in liver transplant candidates found gastric and duodenal portal hypertensive polyposis in 10%

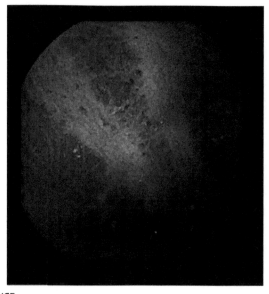

Fig. 4. GAVE on VCE.

and 8%.[32,33] Capsule studies have suggested higher rates of portal hypertension–related polyps, up to 16.3% within the SB.[5] Although these are predominantly found proximally, they can be in any section of the SB, making VCE useful in their investigation.[34] Nevertheless, taking into account technical limitations of VCE (eg, lack of insufflation and irrigation), the diagnosis of these can be difficult, as appearances are often nonspecific and polypoidal lesions in the context of portal hypertension frequently contain ectopic varices. Endoscopic ultrasound (EUS) studies suggest that of the gastric polyps seen endoscopically, 15.8% were ectopic varices, 42.1% had an underlying vessel or varix, and 50% of the lesions thought to be submucosal lesions on EGD were actually varices.[35] As such, very careful assessment, often with EUS, should be considered before polypectomy, and surveillance is often the preferable choice.

SUSPECTED SMALL BOWEL OR OCCULT GASTROINTESTINAL BLEEDING ON THE BACKGROUND OF LIVER DISEASE

Anemia is common in chronic and advanced liver disease, observed in approximately 75% of patients.[36] Causes may be multifactorial, and isolating those who require investigation to identify a bleeding source can be challenging. The liver has a major role in iron homeostasis, making interpretation of iron studies difficult and further to this, iron absorption is impaired, further complicating the clinical picture.[37] When portal hypertensive GI bleeding is suspected, the vast majority are located within the upper GI tract with a smaller, but clinically significant, percentage within the SB.[38] When investigating for occult GI bleeding, liver disease is consistently identified as a factor associated with a high diagnostic yield in VCE.[39,40] In this scenario, angiodysplastic lesions are frequently the most common source.[41,42] Other possible portal hypertension–related findings in the SB are SB varices and portal hypertension enteropathy.

Ectopic varices can be difficult to localize and treat (**Fig. 5**). The prevalence is suggested to be between 6.2% and 8.7%,[41,43,44] and as high as 33.3%.[38] These come

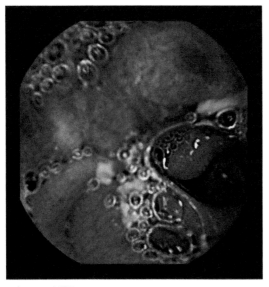

Fig. 5. Ectopic SB varices on VCE.

from small VCE studies or case series and so are hard to generalize but are often thought to be the likely culprit site of bleeding. The prevalence of duodenal varices was 40% in an older series published by Stephan and Miething[45] in those with cirrhosis undergoing angiogram. In a series by Watanabe and colleagues,[46] 32.9% of patients had duodenal varices with 4% in the jejunum and 1.2% in the ileum. Duodenal varices most commonly originate from the inferior pancreaticoduodenal vein, with jejunal or ileal varices arising due to collateralization of the superior and inferior mesenteric veins and retroperitoneal systemic venous systems. On ileocolonoscopy, Misra and colleagues[47] presented ileal varices in 18% with cirrhosis and 0% in those in the control group. VCE in these patients allows noninvasive diagnosis, following which device-assisted enteroscopy may be required to achieve hemostasis.[48] SB vasculopathies, including varices, show improvement or resolution following a transjugular intrahepatic portosystemic shunt procedure,[7] which can be required in recurrent or high-risk bleeding.

Portal hypertensive enteropathy (PHE) encapsulates a wide spectrum of SB changes, from red spots, angioectasia, or inflammatory lesions/polyps. The presence of these changes appears to increase with advancing liver disease and portal pressures, increases in severity with treatment of esophageal varices,[49] and often coexists with other luminal manifestations of portal hypertension. The changes are most pronounced in the proximal and middle SB.[50] In those with mucosal edema exhibiting the classic "herring roe" appearance, there was a strong correlation with increased spleen size and thrombocytopenia.[51] Traditional endoscopy-based studies found a low prevalence of PHE in those with advanced liver disease[47,52] compared with VCE studies, which suggests much higher levels of 57% to 95%.[41,50,53] The most recent studies with the most sensitive technology suggest its presence in more than 95% of those with portal hypertensive changes seen already on either upper or lower GI endoscopy.[5] Possible reasons for this increasing detection may be the improved picture quality allowing for a more sensitive examination, and the lack of air insufflation in VCE allowing subtle mucosal vascular changes to be observed[31] (Video 2).

With increasingly sensitive technology, subtle portal hypertensive changes can be detected, but the clinical significance of these to the individual patient is not always clear. The heterogeneity of patients and their underlying liver disease, presence of PHE even in cirrhotic patients without anemia, as well as the coexistence with mucosal changes in the upper and lower GI tract, make addressing the clinical relevance of SB portal hypertension–related changes problematic (**Table 3**).

Table 3 Summary of possible indications and PH-related findings in chronic liver disease	
Possible Indications of VCE	**PH-Related Findings**
Variceal surveillance	Esophageal varices
	Gastric varices
	Small bowel varices
	Colonic or rectal varices
Iron deficiency anemia	PHG
	GAVE
	PH polyposis
	Angioectasia
	PH gastro/entero/colopathy

Abbreviations: GAVE, gastric antral vascular ectasia; PH, portal hypertension; PHG, portal hypertensive gastropathy.

DISCUSSION AND FUTURE DEVELOPMENTS

Through modification in design, new capsule models are becoming available that allow the physician to focus the examination on specific areas of the GI tract. This has allowed us to examine the esophagus for varices and inspect the SB with a greater degree of accuracy and most recently the possibility of panenteric examination with the introduction of a colon capsule.

Colon capsule has an adaptive frame rate, which alters depending on the speed at which the camera is moving, and an improved battery duration allowing a greater distance to be reached. This, coupled with wide-angle views and 2 camera heads, optimize views of as much mucosa as possible. These technical features allow effective evaluation of the entire GI tract in a single examination. There is a paucity of current literature published on the subject, but in the future, this may be a powerful tool in identifying portal hypertension–related bleeding, such as portal hypertension colopathy or colonic/stomal varices.[54,55] This remains less sensitive than conventional colonoscopy at present, but it is a developing technology and will continue to improve.[56] Panenteric examination through VCE is already viable for the investigation of inflammatory bowel disease[57,58] and could be used in the future for those with cirrhosis in which the colon also could be a source of bleeding. A major limitation in this, however, remains the need for preparation, which can be troublesome even in those without comorbidity.

Current evidence in this area is limited, with guidelines often based on small retrospective studies, but as these technologies become most established, their role in liver disease will become clear.

MACE is suggested to have a higher diagnostic yield in suspected acute upper GI bleeding with better tolerance. It also allows improved visualization of the stomach, which has been a limitation of VCE.[14] By combining gastric and SB investigation, MACE has a higher abnormality detection rate than gastroscopy alone in those with recurrent or refractory iron deficiency anemia.[59] As a technology, this continues to evolve with second-generation MACE allowing improved maneuverability and mucosal visualization.[60]

With the introduction of artificial intelligence in VCE interpretation, it is likely that VCE investigation, as less physician time is required, will become more cost-effective, making it an appealing prospect for those requiring ongoing and often frequent surveillance.[61] VCE is also suggested as a screening tool for liver disease, and although not as sensitive or specific as serologic markers, SB changes were directly proportional to the severity of liver disease.[62]

SUMMARY

In many ways, capsule endoscopy provides suboptimal results when compared with traditional endoscopy for screening or surveillance of esophageal varices, even if specifically modified to improve esophageal mucosa inspection. Upper GI endoscopy is the cornerstone of screening/surveillance programs; however, capsule endoscopy remains a viable alternative in patients unable or unwilling to receive gastroscopy.

SB abnormalities are frequently present in those with liver disease or portal hypertension. Before the invention of VCE, many of these would go undiagnosed but are now accessible, and the clinical significance of many of these findings is often unclear.[5,63]

For several reasons, VCE will not entirely replace the need for invasive procedures in the context of liver disease. Intervention is frequently required, and VCE is a long way from allowing therapy for varices or enteroscopy for SB bleeding, unlike EGD.

Unfortunately, many patients with liver cirrhosis are frail, and avoiding sedation or invasive procedures, which carry significant risk, is appealing. With increasing experience and stepwise evolution of design, VCE continues to improve and widen its role in the field of liver disease.

CLINICS CARE POINTS

- Capsule endoscopy is safe and well tolerated in those with advanced liver disease.
- Capsule endoscopy is a viable option for screening and surveillance of esophageal varices in those unwilling, or unable to tolerate gastroscopy. It is, however, less sensitive.
- Anemia is common in those with liver cirrhosis, and capsule endoscopy frequently defines a cause for this.
- Ongoing advances in capsule design lead to ever-improving detection of panenteric complications of portal hypertension.

DISCLOSURE

A.R. Robertson: nothing to disclose. A. Koulaouzidis: material support for research from SynMed, IntroMedic, and Given Imaging; travel support from Jinshan Technology, Aquiland; advisory consultation(s) from Ankon, IntroMedic; codirector of iCERV and cofounder of AJMMedicaps Ltd. E. Rondonotti: nothing to disclose; Speaker honoraria from Fujifilm Co. M. Bruno: nothing to disclose. M. Pennazio: speaker's fee from Olympus, Medtronic.

SUPPLEMENTARY DATA

Supplementary data related to this article can be found online at https://doi.org/10.1016/j.giec.2020.12.007.

REFERENCES

1. Stokkeland K, Brandt L, Ekbom A, et al. Improved prognosis for patients hospitalized with esophageal varices in Sweden 1969-2002. Hepatology 2006. https://doi.org/10.1002/hep.21089.
2. Turon F, Casu S, Hernández-Gea V, et al. Variceal and other portal hypertension related bleeding. Best Pract Res Clin Gastroenterol 2013. https://doi.org/10.1016/j.bpg.2013.08.004.
3. De Franchis R, Abraldes JG, Bajaj J, et al. Expanding consensus in portal hypertension Report of the Baveno VI Consensus Workshop: Stratifying risk and individualizing care for portal hypertension. J Hepatol 2015. https://doi.org/10.1016/j.jhep.2015.07.001.
4. Seiji K, Akinobu T, Masaya I, et al. Safety and efficacy of small bowel examination by capsule endoscopy for patients before liver transplantation. Biomed Res Int 2017. https://doi.org/10.1155/2017/8193821.
5. Goenka MK, Shah BB, Rai VK, et al. Mucosal changes in the small intestines in portal hypertension: first study using the PillCam SB3 capsule endoscopy system. Clin Endosc 2018. https://doi.org/10.5946/ce.2018.041.
6. Ripoll C, Groszmann R, Garcia-Tsao G, et al. Hepatic venous pressure gradient predicts clinical decompensation in patients with compensated cirrhosis. Gastroenterology 2007. https://doi.org/10.1053/j.gastro.2007.05.024.

7. Matsushita Y, Narahara Y, Fujimori S, et al. Effects of transjugular intrahepatic por-tosystemic shunt on changes in the small bowel mucosa of cirrhotic patients with portal hypertension. J Gastroenterol 2013. https://doi.org/10.1007/s00535-012-0660-6.

8. Al-Azzawi Y, Spaho L, Mahmoud M, et al. Video capsule endoscopy in the assessment of portal hypertensive enteropathy. Int J Hepatol 2018. https://doi.org/10.1155/2018/5109689.

9. Kunihara S, Oka S, Tanaka S, et al. Predictive factors of portal hypertensive en-teropathy exacerbation in patients with liver cirrhosis: a capsule endoscopy study. Digestion 2018. https://doi.org/10.1159/000486666.

10. Abbas N, Makker J, Abbas H, et al. Perioperative care of patients with liver cirrhosis: a review. Heal Serv Insights 2017. https://doi.org/10.1177/1178632917691270.

11. McCarty TR, Afinogenova Y, Njei B. Use of wireless capsule endoscopy for the diagnosis and grading of esophageal varices in patients with portal hypertension: a systematic review and meta-analysis. J Clin Gastroenterol 2017. https://doi.org/10.1097/MCG.0000000000000589.

12. Cardey J, Le Gall C, Michaud L, et al. Screening of esophageal varices in chil-dren using esophageal capsule endoscopy: a multicenter prospective study. Endoscopy 2019. https://doi.org/10.1055/a-0647-1709.

13. Rondonotti E, Spada C, Adler S, et al. Small-bowel capsule endoscopy and device-assisted enteroscopy for diagnosis and treatment of small-bowel disor-ders: European Society of Gastrointestinal Endoscopy (ESGE) Technical Review. Endoscopy 2018. https://doi.org/10.1055/a-0576-0566.

14. Ching HL, Hale MF, Sidhu R, et al. Magnetically assisted capsule endoscopy in suspected acute upper GI bleeding versus esophagogastroduodenoscopy in detecting focal lesions. Gastrointest Endosc 2019. https://doi.org/10.1016/j.gie.2019.04.248.

15. Rondonotti E, Villa F, Dell' Era A, et al. Capsule endoscopy in portal hypertension. Clin Liver Dis 2010. https://doi.org/10.1016/j.cld.2010.03.004.

16. Ramirez FC, Akins R, Shaukat M. Screening of Barrett's esophagus with string-capsule endoscopy: a prospective blinded study of 100 consecutive patients us-ing histology as the criterion standard. Gastrointest Endosc 2008. https://doi.org/10.1016/j.gie.2007.10.040.

17. Liao Z, Gao R, Xu C, et al. Sleeve string capsule endoscopy for real-time viewing of the esophagus: a pilot study (with video). Gastrointest Endosc 2009. https://doi.org/10.1016/j.gie.2008.10.043.

18. Ramirez FC, Hakim S, Tharalson EM, et al. Feasibility and safety of string wireless capsule endoscopy in the diagnosis of esophageal varices. Am J Gastroenterol 2005. https://doi.org/10.1111/j.1572-0241.2005.41037.x.

19. Song J, Bai T, Zhang L, et al. Better view by detachable string magnetically controlled capsule endoscopy for esophageal observation: a retrospective comparative study. Dis Esophagus 2020;33(4):doz104.

20. Chen YZ, Pan J, Luo YY, et al. Detachable string magnetically controlled capsule endoscopy for complete viewing of the esophagus and stomach. Endoscopy 2019. https://doi.org/10.1055/a-0856-6845.

21. Colli A, Gana JC, Turner D, et al. Capsule endoscopy for the diagnosis of oeso-phageal varices in people with chronic liver disease or portal vein thrombosis. Cochrane Database Syst Rev 2014. https://doi.org/10.1002/14651858.CD008760.pub2.

22. Henkel SAF, Squires JE. New tools for screening children with portal hypertension. J Pediatr Gastroenterol Nutr 2019;69(6):639–40.
23. Duché M, Ducot B, Ackermann O, et al. Portal hypertension in children: high-risk varices, primary prophylaxis and consequences of bleeding. J Hepatol 2017. https://doi.org/10.1016/j.jhep.2016.09.006.
24. Pai A, Jonas M, Fox V. Esophageal capsule endoscopy in children and young adults with portal hypertension. J Pediatr Gastroenterol Nutr 2019;69:641–7.
25. Beg S, Card T, Warburton S, et al. Diagnosis of Barrett's esophagus and esophageal varices using a magnetically assisted capsule endoscopy system. Gastrointest Endosc 2020. https://doi.org/10.1016/j.gie.2019.10.031.
26. Krok KL, Wagennar RR, Kantsevoy SV, et al. Esophageal capsule endoscopy is not the optimal technique to determine the need for primary prophylaxis in patients with cirrhosis. Arch Med Sci 2016. https://doi.org/10.5114/aoms.2016.59263.
27. Ching HL, Healy A, Thurston V, et al. Upper gastrointestinal tract capsule endoscopy using a nurse-led protocol: first reported experience. World J Gastroenterol 2018. https://doi.org/10.3748/wjg.v24.i26.2893.
28. Kim MY, Choi H, Baik SK, et al. Portal hypertensive gastropathy: correlation with portal hypertension and prognosis in cirrhosis. Dig Dis Sci 2010. https://doi.org/10.1007/s10620-010-1221-6.
29. D'Amico G, Pagliaro L, Bosch J. The treatment of portal hypertension: a meta-analytic review. Hepatology 1995. https://doi.org/10.1016/0270-9139(95)90388-7.
30. Tekola BD, Caldwell S. Approach to the management of portal hypertensive gastropathy and gastric antral vascular ectasia. Clin Liver Dis 2012. https://doi.org/10.1002/cld.99.
31. Marrero RJ, Barkin JS. Wireless capsule endoscopy and portal hypertensive intestinal vasculopathy. Gastrointest Endosc 2005. https://doi.org/10.1016/j.gie.2005.06.040.
32. Kara D, Hüsing-Kabar A, Schmidt H, et al. Portal hypertensive polyposis in advanced liver cirrhosis: the unknown entity? Can J Gastroenterol Hepatol 2018. https://doi.org/10.1155/2018/2182784.
33. Lemmers A, Evrard S, Demetter P, et al. Gastrointestinal polypoid lesions: a poorly known endoscopic feature of portal hypertension. United Eur Gastroenterol J 2014. https://doi.org/10.1177/2050640614529108.
34. Gurung A. Duodenal polyposis secondary to portal hypertensive duodenopathy. World J Gastrointest Endosc 2015. https://doi.org/10.4253/wjge.v7.i17.1257.
35. Sigounas D, Shams A, Hayes P, et al. Endoscopic ultrasound assessment of gastrointestinal polypoid lesions of indeterminate morphology in patients with portal hypertension. Endosc Int Open 2018. https://doi.org/10.1055/s-0043-124363.
36. McHutchison JG, Manns MP, Longo DL. Definition and management of anemia in patients infected with hepatitis C virus. Liver Int 2006. https://doi.org/10.1111/j.1478-3231.2006.01228.x.
37. Gkamprela E, Deutsch M, Pectasides D. Iron deficiency anemia in chronic liver disease: etiopathogenesis, diagnosis and treatment. Ann Gastroenterol 2017. https://doi.org/10.20524/aog.2017.0152.
38. Akyuz F, Pinarbasi B, Ermis F, et al. Is portal hypertensive enteropathy an important additional cause of blood loss in portal hypertensive patients? Scand J Gastroenterol 2010. https://doi.org/10.3109/00365521.2010.510568.

39. Sidhu R, Sanders DS, Kapur K, et al. Factors predicting the diagnostic yield and intervention in obscure gastrointestinal bleeding investigated using capsule endoscopy. J Gastrointest Liver Dis 2009;18(3):273–8.

40. Carey EJ, Leighton JA, Heigh RI, et al. A single-center experience of 260 consecutive patients undergoing capsule endoscopy for obscure gastrointestinal bleeding. Am J Gastroenterol 2007. https://doi.org/10.1111/j.1572-0241.2006.00941.x.

41. De Palma GD, Rega M, Masone S, et al. Mucosal abnormalities of the small bowel in patients with cirrhosis and portal hypertension: a capsule endoscopy study. Gastrointest Endosc 2005. https://doi.org/10.1016/S0016-5107(05)01588-9.

42. Yamada A, Watabe H, Obi S, et al. Surveillance of small intestinal abnormalities in patients with hepatocellular carcinoma: a prospective capsule endoscopy study. Dig Endosc 2011. https://doi.org/10.1111/j.1443-1661.2010.01050.x.

43. Chandrasekar TS, Janakan GB, Chandrasekar VT, et al. Spectrum of small-bowel mucosal abnormalities identified by capsule endoscopy in patients with portal hypertension of varied etiology. Indian J Gastroenterol 2017. https://doi.org/10.1007/s12664-016-0721-5.

44. Tang SJ, Zanati S, Dubcenco E, et al. Diagnosis of small-bowel varices by capsule endoscopy. Gastrointest Endosc 2004. https://doi.org/10.1016/S0016-5107(04)01458-0.

45. Stephan G, Miething R. Rontgendiagnostik varicoser duodenal veranderungen bei portaler hypertension. Der Radiol 1968;8(3):90–5.

46. Watanabe N, Toyonaga A, Kojima S, et al. Current status of ectopic varices in Japan: results of a survey by the Japan Society for Portal Hypertension. Hepatol Res 2010. https://doi.org/10.1111/j.1872-034X.2010.00690.x.

47. Misra SP, Dwivedi M, Misra V, et al. Ileal varices and portal hypertensive ileopathy in patients with cirrhosis and portal hypertension. Gastrointest Endosc 2004. https://doi.org/10.1016/S0016-5107(04)02049-8.

48. Despott EJ, May A, Lazaridis N, et al. Double-balloon enteroscopy–facilitated cyanoacrylate-injection endotherapy of small-bowel varices: an international experience from 2 European tertiary centers (with videos). Gastrointest Endosc 2019. https://doi.org/10.1016/j.gie.2019.03.1171.

49. Otani I, Oka S, Aikata H, et al. Exacerbation of portal hypertensive enteropathy after endoscopic injection sclerotherapy for esophageal varices. Digestion 2019. https://doi.org/10.1159/000503060.

50. Aoyama T, Oka S, Aikata H, et al. Major predictors of portal hypertensive enteropathy in patients with liver cirrhosis. J Gastroenterol Hepatol 2015. https://doi.org/10.1111/jgh.12658.

51. Higaki N, Matsui H, Imaoka H, et al. Characteristic endoscopic features of portal hypertensive enteropathy. J Gastroenterol 2008. https://doi.org/10.1007/s00535-008-2166-9.

52. Desai N, Desai D, Pethe V, et al. Portal hypertensive jejunopathy: a case control study. Indian J Gastroenterol 2004;23(3):99–101.

53. Dabos KJ, Yung DE, Bartzis L, et al. Small bowel capsule endoscopy and portal hypertensive enteropathy in cirrhotic patients: results from a tertiary referral centre. Ann Hepatol 2016. https://doi.org/10.5604/16652681.1198815.

54. Hong SN, Kang SH, Jang HJ, et al. Recent advance in colon capsule endoscopy: what's new? Clin Endosc 2018. https://doi.org/10.5946/ce.2018.121.

55. Kawasaki K, Kakisaka K, Matsumoto T. Idiopathic ileocolonic varices depicted by colon capsule endoscopy. Dig Endosc 2016. https://doi.org/10.1111/den.12660.

56. Van Gossum A, Navas MM, Fernandez-Urien I, et al. Capsule endoscopy versus colonoscopy for the detection of polyps and cancer. N Engl J Med 2009. https://doi.org/10.1056/NEJMoa0806347.

57. Tai D, Thurston V, Healy A, et al. First clinical experience of panenteric capsule endoscopy using the PillCam Crohn's capsule. Gut 2018. https://doi.org/10.1136/gutjnl-2018-BSGAbstracts.194.

58. Eliakim R, Spada C, Lapidus A, et al. Evaluation of a new pan-enteric video capsule endoscopy system in patients with suspected or established inflammatory bowel disease – feasibility study. Endosc Int Open 2018. https://doi.org/10.1055/a-0677-170.

59. Ching HL, Hale MF, Sidhu R, et al. Capsule endoscopy has better diagnostic yield than gastroscopy in recurrent iron deficiency anaemia. Gut 2018. https://doi.org/10.1136/gutjnl-2018-BSGAbstracts.21.

60. Jiang B, Qian Y-Y, Pan J, et al. Second-generation magnetically controlled capsule gastroscopy with improved image resolution and frame rate: a randomized controlled clinical trial (with video). Gastrointest Endosc 2020;91(6):1379–87.

61. Le Berre C, Sandborn WJ, Aridhi S, et al. Application of artificial intelligence to gastroenterology and hepatology. Gastroenterology 2020. https://doi.org/10.1053/j.gastro.2019.08.058.

62. Wu L-H, Chen M-H, Cai J-Y, et al. The correlation between intestinal mucosal lesions and hepatic dysfunction in patients without chronic liver disease. Medicine (Baltimore) 2020;7(99):e18837.

63. Urbain D, Vandebosch S, Hindryckx P, et al. Capsule endoscopy findings in cirrhosis with portal hypertension: a prospective study. Dig Liver Dis 2008. https://doi.org/10.1016/j.dld.2007.12.015.

Video Capsule Endoscopy Beyond the Gastrointestinal Suite

Joel Lange, MD[a], Arooj Shah, MD[b], Andrew C. Meltzer, MD, MS[a],*

KEYWORDS

- Video capsule endoscopy • Pillcam • Capsule endoscopy • Endoscopy
- GI bleeding • Emergency department

KEY POINTS

- Video capsule endoscopy (VCE) has been used for diagnosing diseases of the gastrointestinal (GI) tract and as an alternative modality to traditional endoscopy.
- In settings such as the emergency room, the intensive care unit, and outpatient settings, VCE might be the only feasible tool to assess and visualize the GI tract.
- Research is ongoing to determine if more widespread use is safe, effective and feasible.

INTRODUCTION

Video capsule endoscopy (VCE) was first described by Iddan and colleagues[1] in 2000 as a novel means to remotely view the lumen of the gastrointestinal (GI) tract. Early adaptors foresaw a revolutionary tool that might replace some of the functions of traditional tube-based endoscopy, the bedrock of modern gastroenterology. The potential advantages of VCE include that it can be administered by a nonspecialist, without anesthesia, and, in any clinical setting. Subsequent studies described high patient tolerance and accuracy levels similar to traditional esophagogastroduodenoscopy (EGD).[2-5] Over time, VCE has gained acceptance as an alternative modality for identifying mucosal lesions, assessing gastric motility and diagnosing inflammatory bowel disease.[2,3,6-8] However, it has never approached the early promise of replacing traditional endoscopy. For most gastroenterologists, traditional endoscopy is preferred due to the ability to manipulate the image, perform a biopsy, provide hemostatic therapy, insufflate the lumen, and earn higher reimbursement. Yet, the use of VCE in nontraditional

a Department of Emergency Medicine, George Washington University School of Medicine and Health Sciences, 2120 L Street Northwest, Suite 450, Washington, DC 20037, USA; b Department of Emergency Medicine, George Washington Medical Faculty Associates, 2120 L Street Northwest, Suite 450, Washington, DC 20037, USA
* Corresponding author.
E-mail address: ameltzer@mfa.gwu.edu

Gastrointest Endoscopy Clin N Am 31 (2021) 377–385
https://doi.org/10.1016/j.giec.2020.12.005
1052-5157/21/© 2020 Elsevier Inc. All rights reserved.

endoscopic settings is slowly gaining a permanent hold. In settings such as the emergency room (ER), the intensive care unit (ICU), the office practice, or urgent care, VCE may represent the only feasible tool to view the gastrointestinal lumen. In this review, we explore the diverse uses of VCE in variety of novel settings.

NOVEL SETTINGS FOR VIDEO CAPSULE ENDOSCOPY
Intensive Care Unit

The use of endoscopic procedures may be limited due to the health of the patient. Patients will often require sedation measures for their procedure, which may not be feasible for very sick patients. The less invasive nature of VCE may make it preferable in certain situations in the ICU. Boutros and colleagues[9] retrospectively reviewed all capsule endoscopy studies performed in their medical ICU for the purposes of investigating obscure gastrointestinal bleeds requiring multiple transfusions. The study included a total of 12 patients, of whom 8 (66%) of 12 had a significant finding that may explain the patient's bleeding. Limitations encountered in the ICU include the inability to swallow, mechanical ventilation, and altered intestinal motility. A hybrid model of endoscopy in which the EGD places the VCE in a post-pyloric position may further be beneficial for the ICU population.

Perioperative Video Capsule Endoscopy

VCE has been proposed and used as a modality to investigate GI bleeding before proceeding to the operating room, specifically for planning for treating suspected small bowel bleeding that cannot be managed enteroscopically. Before the advent of VCE, the primary modalities of diagnosing small bowel pathology was radiologic (small bowel follow-through, radionucleotide, or angiography), endoscopy (push endoscopy, intraoperative endoscopy, or deep enteroscopy), or via surgical investigation. These modalities were limited by the invasive nature of the procedure, the inability to detect a lesion without active bleeding, and the inability to reach the site of the bleeding.[10] Ersoy and colleagues[10] first described the applicability of VCE visualization of bleeding sources, tumors, diffuse mucosal pathologies (Crohn disease, ulcerative colitis) and atrioventricular malformations as an alternative modality for preoperative planning. The advantages to the surgeon are an accurate modality for bowel visualization that is less invasive than many others.

Vere and colleagues[11] further evaluated the use of VCE in investigating small bowel tumor pathology for surgical intervention perioperatively. The 2012 report investigated 50 patients presenting with signs of GI bleeding (eg, hematochezia, blood in stool) using VCE, of whom 11 had visualization of a small bowel tumor, which was the primary modality for establishing a surgically addressable lesion. The patients then underwent surgery with 10 (91%) of 11 having surgical resection performed on the visualized site.

Hemodialysis

VCE has shown promise by allowing for less invasive investigation of chronically ill patients with kidney failure. A higher prevalence of bowel pathology in patients with end-stage renal disease (ESRD) than the general population has been previously reported.[12,13] However, due to the greater disease burden of patients with ESRD, they may have limited access to endoscopy and other invasive diagnostic procedures. Hosoe and colleagues[14] performed VCE on 54 patients with ESRD who received maintenance hemodialysis 3 times per week. In 65% of participants, small bowel lesions were detected, and, of these, 39% had mucosal lesions, 19% had vascular lesions, and 7% had both.[14,15] Because hemodialysis requires several hours per session and multiple sessions per week, the work flow with administering VCE seems feasible as a program that could be expanded.

Emergency Room

An EGD is rarely performed in the ER itself because of the need for a gastroenterologist, for specialized equipment, and, for anesthesia support. Because of these barriers, patients with severe lesions may receive delayed care and patients with benign or trivial lesions may receive an unnecessary hospital admission. Current tools to perform risk stratification have significant limitations involving accuracy or efficiency including the Glasgow-Blatchford score, nasogastric (NG) lavage, or the "admit-all" strategy. The use of VCE could allow an emergency physician to examine the lumen of the GI tract at the bedside to identify the presence or absence of an active bleed or high-risk lesion and serve as more accurate risk stratification tool.

Multiple studies have investigated this scenario. Rubin and colleagues[16] described how VCE could be used for risk stratification in identifying patients who require urgent endoscopy and therapeutic intervention. In this study, 24 patients were randomized to either VCE or standard clinical assessment. Patients with positive VCE findings for upper gastrointestinal bleeding (UGIB) were directed to have urgent EGD within 6 hours, thereby reducing time to EGD; however, the requirement of blood transfusion and mortality were not affected.[16] Meltzer and colleagues[17] in 2012 described the use of VCE to detect bleeding in the ER in a study of 25 patients with suspected UGIB. In this study, VCE was 88% sensitive to detect an acute UGIB and there was good agreement in the detection of an UGIB between reading emergency physicians and gastroenterologists. Gralnek and colleagues in 2013 performed a randomized clinical trial on the use of VCE for initial evaluation of patients with acute UGIB compared with NG tube or to an EGD (Available at: http://www.thieme-connect.com/products/ejournals/abstract/10.1055/s-0032-1325933). The researchers reported significantly more identification of UGIB in the VCE versus the NG aspiration method (83.3% vs 33.3%) despite no significant difference in lesion detection.[18] Gutkin and colleagues[19] in 2013 compared the use of PillCam ESO against the Rockall and Blatchford scoring systems for identifying high-risk patients with UGIB in 24 patients presenting to a single ER. Twelve patients had a VCE, of whom 8 of 12 had findings concerning for a high-risk UGIB which were confirmed on subsequent EGD. The 4 of 12 patients without significant VCE findings all had negative results on subsequent EGD. The Rockall and Blatchford scores for the 24 patients in the study were not statistically different whether they had high-risk or low-risk findings on their EGD. Finally, Sung and colleagues[20] performed a prospective randomized controlled trial to determine if VCE could safely decrease hospital admissions. For patients who presented with signs and symptoms of UGIB, 7 (19%) of 37 patients randomized to the VCE group were admitted to the hospital, versus 34 (100%) of 34 patients in the standard treatment group. However, there was no difference in recurrent bleeding, or 30-day mortality.[20]

One study examined the use of VCE for nonspecific chest pain in the ER. Millions of people present annually to the ER in the United States with chest pain, and only a minority of these patients have cardiac disease. Singh et al[21] conducted a pilot study in which they used PillCam ESO in patients presenting to the ER with noncardiac chest pain after Acute Coronary Syndrome (ACS) was ruled out. In this study, 44% of participants were found to have esophageal mucosal abnormalities, 40% had erosive esophagitis, and 4% were found to show mucosal changes consistent with Barrett esophagus (BE).

Out-of-Clinic Settings

VCE may play an important role in both rural and isolated locations or in settings such as correctional facilities where transportation is challenging. Adler and colleagues[22] described the use of VCE to image the colon in lieu of a traditional colonoscopy in a geographically isolated setting, where patients had to travel more than 40 minutes to get to a GI procedural clinic. In this study of 41 patients, VCE was used for colorectal cancer screening (78%), investigating the source of a GI bleed (10%), surveillance of inflammatory bowel disease (5%), an abnormal computed tomography scan (5%), and surveillance in the setting of familial colorectal cancer history (2%).[22] Examinations were complete and successful for imaging acquisition in 88% of patients and lesions detected were generally confirmed by subsequent colonoscopies.[22] VCE image transmission could allow rural primary physicians to order VCE studies and have expert review. Therefore, using VCE as a visualization method in circumstances in which traditional modalities are challenging to perform is a promising approach by allowing for more widespread and expert access, particularly when in geographic isolation/rural settings.

NON-GASTROENTEROLOGISTS AS VIDEO CAPSULE ENDOSCOPY INTERPRETERS
Training with Video Capsule Endoscopy

The American Society of Gastrointestinal Endoscopy (ASGE) published guidelines on the development of a curriculum for small bowel endoscopy in the setting of gastroenterology fellowships.[23] At least 20 supervised procedures were recommended for providers planning to practice VCE independently and they recommended a greater than 90% ability to identify significant pathologic findings on VCE on a formalized in-service examination or when compared with a credentialed endoscopist. In addition, a fellowship program is recommended to have at least 1 certified capsule endoscopist on staff in the program and have sufficient volume to give fellows sufficient exposure to VCE (at least 20). As of 2018, most GI training programs had formal VCE training incorporated into their curriculums.[24] For non-gastroenterologist physicians or non-physician providers, there is also a need to validate training. For other providers, it remains possible to take courses sponsored by the ASGE to substitute for formal training.[23,25]

Emergency Physicians

It is unknown if the accuracy between emergency physicians and gastroenterologists for interpreting blood on VCE is similar. Due to the time-sensitive nature of UGIB and the lack of GI clinicians on an emergency 24/7 basis, the question of whether a non-GI specialist such as an ER doctor can detect GI bleeding with VCE is important. Meltzer and colleagues[26] conducted a survey study in 2013 in which they showed video clips of ED patients with GI bleeding after a brief 15-minute training session. For 126 emergency medicine resident or attending physicians without prior endoscopy training, there was sensitivity of 0.94 and specificity of 0.87 of physicians to identify the presence or absence of GI bleeding compared with a gold standard read.[26]

Nurse Protocols

A major limitation of VCE has been the time-consuming nature of reviewing images captured by the capsule and camera. A normal capsule endoscopic procedure can result in thousands of images, any one of which may contain a lesion. It takes an average of 50 minutes for a physician to view all the images from a small bowel

VCE.[27] Using specialized nurses for providing initial interpretation of the studies has been studied as a more cost-effective and efficient approach. In general, nurses are trained to detect possible lesions and then physicians look at any suspected abnormalities. In one study, the endoscopy nurse had a 93% sensitivity of detecting lesions seen by gastroenterologists.[27] In another study, Bossa and colleagues[28] reported on the degree of agreement between an endoscopy nurse and an endoscopist. There was high level agreement for certain lesions such as active bleeding and stenosis (kappa >0.85), but there was moderate agreement for more subtle nonpathologic mucosal abnormalities (kappa = 0.77).[28]

Artificial Intelligence–Assisted Protocols

To address the labor and time-intensive issues surrounding VCE, artificial intelligence (AI) and computer-aided diagnostic strategies have been undertaken by several investigators. There have been several reports that have identified the ability for AI to detect lesions, and researchers have reported a reduction in the time required for total study review.[29–32]

One early challenge that needed to be addressed by AI was identifying where a VCE was physically located at any given time during the study. Zou and colleagues[33] in 2015 used AI to identify and classify portions of the digestive tract (stomach, small intestine, or large intestine) with VCE images. They investigated more than 60,000 training images collected from 25 patients and noted an accuracy of 95.5% for correct identification of the anatomic region.[33]

AI has also been studied regarding the ability to need to accurately and readily identify sources of bleeding or hemorrhage in patients. Xiao and Meng[34] in 2016 and later Li and colleagues[35] in 2017 reported the development a strategy to detect bleeding sources and active hemorrhages within AI. They developed strategies that were able to correctly identify a source of bleeding with an accuracy of greater than 99% and 100%, respectively, and sensitivities of 99.2% and 98.7%, respectively.[34,35] Leenhardt and colleagues[29] developed a computer-assisted diagnostic tool for detection of angioectasias with a sensitivity of 100% and a specificity of 96% with a positive predictive value of 96% and negative predictive value of 100%. Finally, AI has also been investigated as a modality of identifying polyps seen on VCE studies. Yuan and Meng[36] in 2017 used AI to identify polyps seen during VCE investigations with an accuracy of 98%.

INNOVATIVE APPLICATIONS OF VIDEO CAPSULE ENDOSCOPY
Chronic Diarrhea

Finding the etiology of chronic diarrhea, defined as diarrhea that lasts more than 2 weeks, is challenging. Endoscopic methods have often been used as a modality of investigation with mixed results. Song and colleagues[37] performed a retrospective analysis of 91 patients with chronic diarrhea who received a VCE. This study demonstrated a positive diagnostic yield in 43% of participants. In the patients who underwent VCE, 20% had erosions/aphthous ulcers, 18% had ulcers, 3% had mucosal erythema, 1% had edema, and 1% had luminal narrowing.[37] As a result of the study, 34.1% of patients had a change in their diagnosis from chronic diarrhea to another diagnoses, including irritable bowel syndrome, suspected Crohn disease, or others. This study indicated a new and nontraditional modality for further investigation of chronic problems that is well tolerated by patients with a relatively high diagnostic yield.

Obesity

VCE has also been proposed for management of obesity. Do and colleagues[38] described the proposed use of an ingestible intragastric balloon that has inflatable functions for the use of a structural weight loss modality. Using this device, patients swallow a capsule that inflates in the gastric space to induce the feeling of satiety. When the balloon is to be removed, it can simply be deflated and passed. The design still requires validation, but is a promising and novel concept for a potentially easier and safer bariatric alternative to surgery.

COST/COST-EFFECTIVENESS

One of the major limitations of traditional endoscopic procedures is the resource-intensive nature of performing such an invasive procedure. Several clinicians have proposed that VCE may be able to provide an alternative and less costly modality of visualizing the gastrointestinal tract. Traditional endoscopic methods have high financial burdens to patients and society because of the costs associated with the physician performing the endoscopy, the costs of the facility being used/staff of that facility, and the costs of anesthesia (including anesthesiologist, anesthetic drugs, and postanesthesia monitoring). VCE has the advantage of allowing any provider or nurse to administer the test and then a subsequent VCE-trained provider to interpret the images.

Patients with Crohn disease have a high financial burden for disease maintenance due in large part to the recurring need for direct visualizing procedures. Lobo and colleagues[39] evaluated the cost-saving measures that could be incurred by incorporating VCE in lieu of regular visualizing procedures, colonoscopies coupled with magnetic resonance enterography (MRE). The analysis showed increased quality adjusted life years with VCE versus colonoscopy ± MRE (10.67 vs 10.97 years) and decreased 20-year cost by almost 10% (£42,266 vs £38,043).[39]

Researchers have also proposed using VCE as a modality to reduce the need for EGDs in diagnosing BE. Lin and colleagues[40] tested VCE as a screening method, and then performed EGDs on patients with concerning findings on those examinations. The researchers reported a 67% sensitivity and 84% specificity for identifying BE, yielding positive predictive values and negative predictive values of 22% and 98%, respectively. The researchers therefore described only moderate sensitivity and specificity for identifying BE and therefore not acceptable as a modality for primary screening.[41] Future studies with updated technology may need to revisit this application.

Meltzer and colleagues in 2013[42,43] performed a cost-effective analysis comparing multiple strategies to risk stratify ED patients with UGIB. The 4 strategies considered were (1) VCE in the ED, (2) Glasgow-Blatchford score, (3) NG aspiration, and (4) admit-all strategy. In this study, VCE was equal or superior to other strategies in low to moderate-risk patients but had no effect on cost-effectiveness in high-risk groups. In summary, if VCE can save a hospital admission, the test is cost-effective despite the increased upfront costs.

SUMMARY

Although VCE is well-established for inspection of the small bowel, it has not supplanted EGD or colonoscopy in traditional GI investigations. However, in nontraditional settings, such as the ER and ICU, and with non-gastroenterologist providers, VCE remains poised to be a disruptive innovation in the diagnosis of GI disorders.

CLINICS CARE POINTS

- Video Capsule Endoscopy has been shown to be a sensitive means to detect upper GI bleeding in the ER.
- VCE has diagnostic capability and is unable to provide therapy to stop bleeding.

REFERENCES

1. Iddan G, Meron G, Glukhovsky A, et al. Wireless capsule endoscopy. Nature 2000;405(6785):417.
2. McAlindon ME, Ching HL, Yung D, et al. Capsule endoscopy of the small bowel. Ann Transl Med 2016;4(19):369.
3. Koulaouzidis A, Iakovidis DK, Karargyris A, et al. Optimizing lesion detection in small-bowel capsule endoscopy: from present problems to future solutions. Expert Rev Gastroenterol Hepatol 2015;9(2):217–35.
4. Wong RF, Tuteja AK, Haslem DS, et al. Video capsule endoscopy compared with standard endoscopy for the evaluation of small-bowel polyps in persons with familial adenomatous polyposis (with video). Gastrointest Endosc 2006;64(4): 530–7.
5. Choi M, Lim S, Choi MG, et al. Effectiveness of capsule endoscopy compared with other diagnostic modalities in patients with small bowel Crohn's disease: a meta-analysis. Gut Liver 2017;11(1):62–72.
6. Liao Z, Gao R, Xu C, et al. Indications and detection, completion, and retention rates of small-bowel capsule endoscopy: a systematic review. Gastrointest Endosc 2010;71(2):280–6.
7. Ell C, Remke S, May A, et al. The first prospective controlled trial comparing wireless capsule endoscopy with push enteroscopy in chronic gastrointestinal bleeding. Endoscopy 2002;34(9):685–9.
8. Hejazi RA, Bashashati M, Saadi M, et al. Video capsule endoscopy: a tool for the assessment of small bowel transit time. Front Med (Lausanne) 2016;3:6.
9. Small-bowel capsule endoscopy for obscure gastrointestinal bleeding in the ICU. PMID: 30617592 https://doi.org/10.1007/s00134-018-05506-9.
10. Ersoy O, Sivri B, Bayraktar Y. How helpful is capsule endoscopy to surgeons? World J Gastroenterol 2007;13(27):3671–6.
11. Vere CC, Streba CT, Rogoveanu I, et al. The contribution of the video capsule endoscopy in establishing the indication of surgical treatment in the tumoral pathology of the small bowel. Curr Health Sci J 2012;38(2):69–73.
12. Etemad B. Gastrointestinal complications of renal failure. Gastroenterol Clin North Am 1998;27(4):875–92.
13. Luo J, Leu H, Hou M, et al. Nonpeptic ulcer, nonvariceal gastrointestinal bleeding in hemodialysis patients. Am J Med 2013;126(3):264.e25–32.
14. Hosoe N, Matsukawa S, Kanno Y, et al. Cross-sectional small intestinal surveillance of maintenance hemodialysis patients using video capsule endoscopy: SCHEMA study. Endosc Int Open 2016;4(5):589.
15. Ichikawa R, Hosoe N, Imaeda H, et al. Evaluation of small-intestinal abnormalities in adult patients with henoch-schonlein purpura using video capsule. Endoscopy 2011;43(Suppl 2 UCTN):162.
16. Rubin M, Hussain SA, Shalomov A, et al. Live view video capsule endoscopy enables risk stratification of patients with acute upper GI bleeding in the emergency room: a pilot study. Dig Dis Sci 2011;56(3):786–91.

17. Meltzer AC, Ali MA, Kresiberg RB, et al. Video capsule endoscopy in the emergency department: A prospective study of acute upper gastrointestinal hemorrhage. Ann Emerg Med 2013;61(4):438–43.e1.

18. Klein A, Gralnek IM. Video capsule endoscopy for triage of patients with acute upper GI hemorrhage: is seeing believing? Gastrointest Endosc 2016;84(6): 914–6.

19. Gutkin E, Shalomov A, Hussain SA, et al. Pillcam ESO((R)) is more accurate than clinical scoring systems in risk stratifying emergency room patients with acute upper gastrointestinal bleeding. Therap Adv Gastroenterol 2013;6(3):193–8.

20. Sung JJY, Tang RSY, Ching JYL, et al. Use of capsule endoscopy in the emergency department as a triage of patients with GI bleeding. Gastrointest Endosc 2016;84(6):907–13.

21. Available at: https://d1wqtxts1xzle7.cloudfront.net/50410163/S0016-5085_2810_
2963083-120161118-22748-orio3y.pdf?1479535661=&response-content-
disposition=inline%3B+filename%3DW1189_Influence_of_Simeticone_and_
Metocl.pdf&Expires=1608743457&Signature=MPPi9eZ~HdEuxiJBLFtIJArx
AjJmI4HxEnxTtcSJssWBPz2wJ4ufVGHYo2O4Vq57yss7SJ-klOI4I-QkLizflmQB8
M4EzFTyqVeG6Kelt-rntk1eouPD4gjEfUYhWhZnoTJAH3OJsFzu8GyDpip8ZbJv7
ULJ7YstoFW-M2ERFG32jhfL3lpLdKxwAEHf3mHTdFhQfVGPTsxfF9mqGjOBE
DnF3q6VjVm5m2xZGxmMedPOMOdKuKKq5dPGlXc7YIe36rsHKDzivrjTOYObO
UGuyI2CeRAfa8PaUS41Ez4pjt1gCi6uF9g7zaNBczS-3GwZnx5ukTArT62jj~bo
WtG5FA__&Key-Pair-Id=APKAJLOHF5GGSLRBV4ZA.

22. Adler SN, Hassan C, Metzger Y, et al. Second-generation colon capsule endoscopy is feasible in the out-of-clinic setting. Surg Endosc 2014;28(2):570–5.

23. ASGE Training Committee 2011-2012, Rajan EA, Pais SA, et al. Small-bowel endoscopy core curriculum. Gastrointest Endosc 2013;77(1):1–6.

24. Read AJ, Rice MD, Conjeevaram HS, et al. A deeper look at the small bowel: training pathways in video capsule endoscopy and device-assisted enteroscopy. Dig Dis Sci 2018;63(9):2210–9.

25. Faigel DO, Baron TH, Adler DG, et al. ASGE guideline: guidelines for credentialing and granting privileges for capsule endoscopy. Gastrointest Endosc 2005; 61(4):503–5.

26. Meltzer AC, Pinchbeck C, Burnett S, et al. Emergency physicians accurately interpret video capsule endoscopy findings in suspected upper gastrointestinal hemorrhage: a video survey. Acad Emerg Med 2013;20(7):711–5.

27. Levinthal GN, Burke CA, Santisi JM. The accuracy of an endoscopy nurse in interpreting capsule endoscopy. Am J Gastroenterol 2003;98(12):2669–71.

28. Bossa F, Cocomazzi G, Valvano MR, et al. Detection of abnormal lesions recorded by capsule endoscopy. A prospective study comparing endoscopist's and nurse's accuracy. Dig Liver Dis 2006;38(8):599–602.

29. Leenhardt R, Vasseur P, Li C, et al. A neural network algorithm for detection of GI angiectasia during small-bowel capsule endoscopy. Gastrointest Endosc 2019; 89(1):189–94.

30. Pogorelov K, Suman S, Azmadi Hussin F, et al. Bleeding detection in wireless capsule endoscopy videos - color versus texture features. J Appl Clin Med Phys 2019;20(8):141–54.

31. Iakovidis DK, Koulaouzidis A. Automatic lesion detection in capsule endoscopy based on color saliency: Closer to an essential adjunct for reviewing software. Gastrointest Endosc 2014;80(5):877–83.

32. Pan G, Yan G, Qiu X, et al. Bleeding detection in wireless capsule endoscopy based on probabilistic neural network. J Med Syst 2011;35(6):1477–84.

33. Zou Y, Li L, Wang Y, et al. Classifying digestive organs in wireless capsule endos-copy images based on deep convolutional neural network. Int Conf Digit Signal Process Proc 2015;2015:1274–8.
34. Xiao J, Meng MQ. A deep convolutional neural network for bleeding detection in wireless capsule endoscopy images. Annu Int Conf IEEE Eng Med Biol Soc 2016; 2016:639–42.
35. Li P, Li Z, Gao F, et al. Convolutional neural networks for intestinal hemorrhage detection in wireless capsule endoscopy images. IEEE Int Conf Multimed Expo 2017;2017:1518–23.
36. Yuan Y, Meng MQ. Deep learning for polyp recognition in wireless capsule endoscopy images. Med Phys 2017;44(4):1379–89.
37. Song HJ, Moon JS, Jeon SR, et al. Diagnostic yield and clinical impact of video capsule endoscopy in patients with chronic diarrhea: a Korean multicenter CA-PENTRY study. Gut Liver 2017;11(2):253–60.
38. Do TN, Seah TE, Ho KY, et al. Correction: Development and testing of a magnet-ically actuated capsule endoscopy for obesity treatment. PLoS One 2016;11(3): e0151711.
39. Lobo A, Torrejon Torres R, McAlindon M, et al. Economic analysis of the adoption of capsule endoscopy within the British NHS. Int J Qual Health Care 2020;32(5): 332–41.
40. Lin OS, Schembre DB, Mergener K, et al. Blinded comparison of esophageal capsule endoscopy versus conventional endoscopy for a diagnosis of Barrett's esophagus in patients with chronic gastroesophageal reflux. Gastrointest Endosc 2007;65(4):577–83.
41. Gerson L, Lin OS. Cost-benefit analysis of capsule endoscopy compared with standard upper endoscopy for the detection of Barrett's esophagus. Clin Gastro-enterol Hepatol 2007;5(3):319–25.
42. Meltzer AC, Ward MJ, Gralnek IM, et al. The cost-effectiveness analysis of video capsule endoscopy compared to other strategies to manage acute upper gastro-intestinal hemorrhage in the ED. Am J Emerg Med 2014;32(8):823–32.
43. Blatchford O, Murray WR, Blatchford M. A risk score to predict need for treatment for upper gastrointestinal haemorrhage. Lancet 2000;356(9238):1318–21.

Artificial Intelligence Research and Development for Application in Video Capsule Endoscopy

Peter Sullivan, MD, Shradha Gupta, MD, Patrick D. Powers, Neil B. Marya, MD*

KEYWORDS

- Artificial intelligence • Deep learning • Machine learning
- Convolutional neural networks • Video capsule endoscopy

KEY POINTS

- Video capsule endoscopy is an ideal platform for the development of Artificial Intelligence research.
- Advancements in computer processing capabilities now allow for the development of deep learning models, such as convolutional neural networks, which are capable of autonomous learning when provided large data sets.
- Deep learning models using video capsule endoscopy as a platform have been developed for a wide range of pathologic conditions.

INTRODUCTION

Research into the development of artificial intelligence (AI) applications for medicine has expanded rapidly over the past decade, and AI is increasingly accepted and widely used in medicine, such as improving the precision of diagnostic procedures, refining the accuracy of disease prognoses, and automating documentation.

Although the foundation and first embodiments of modern AI were developed in the 1950s, most formal definitions of AI are loose, and tests (like the epochal Turing test) are subjective in some way, ultimately requiring human assessments of a machine's perceived intelligence. Because of the remarkable contemporary attention to applied AI in industry, research, and elsewhere, the waters are quickly muddied on what AI is or how it can be used. Broadly, modern AI applications in medicine can be labeled "narrow" AIs, which consist of focused decision making or prediction processes for

Division of Gastroenterology, University of Massachusetts Medical School, 55 Lake Avenue North, Worcester, MA 01655, USA
* Corresponding author.
E-mail address: neil.marya@umassmed.edu

Gastrointest Endoscopy Clin N Am 31 (2021) 387–397
https://doi.org/10.1016/j.giec.2020.12.009
giendo.theclinics.com

strictly defined problems, such as predicting if a lesion is present in a digital image, or if the lesion is malignant.

Because AI is a decision-making or prediction process, similar to flipping a coin or linear regression, myriad AI approaches exist and new ones are under constant development, each tailored to specific needs: decision-making quality, speed of a prediction, hardware requirements such as limited memory, processing power, and cost, can all dictate an AI architecture. Artificial neural network (ANN) models are 1 class of AI architectures, also dating to the 1950s, but their potential performance, inspired by the deep biological neural networks in nature, was long restricted by hardware constraints. However, as computational power and affordability have improved in this century, ANNs with highly performant architectures, specifically convolutional neural network (CNN) models, are able to combine great network depth with technical feasibility and are capable of learning to identify sophisticated features from data to make effective decisions in many domains, especially those rich in image data.

Across medicine, clinicians have applied CNN models to analyze mammograms, histopathology slides, electrocardiograms, and fundic retinographies.[1-5] Within gastroenterology, there are several opportunities for CNN models to aid in clinical practice given the range of endoscopic procedures and imaging studies performed for lesion detection and classification.

Perhaps the most notable application within gastroenterology thus far is the development of CNNs for detection and classification of polyps during colonoscopy. A recent study by Urban and colleagues[6] used deep learning to identify and localize polyps during screening colonoscopies in real time. This study included more than 2000 patients and more than 8500 images of polyps to train a CNN model. The investigators found that their model was able to identify polyps with a 96% accuracy rate. Another study, by Zachariah and colleagues, [7] involved a CNN-based optical pathologic condition model to classify colorectal polyps during colonoscopies. This system was able to predict polyp pathologic condition as either adenomas or hyperplastic polyps with an overall accuracy rate of 94%.

Beyond colonoscopy, other potential areas of focus for AI development in gastroenterology and hepatology include pancreatic cancer, hepatocellular carcinoma, gastric cancer, and cirrhosis.[8] Researchers have already developed CNNs that can distinguish focal chronic pancreatitis from pancreatic ductal adenocarcinoma based on endoscopic ultrasound–elastography as well as models that can accurately diagnose liver fibrosis and chronic liver disease.[9,10] Perhaps the most fertile territory for endoscopic CNN development has been databases comprising video capsule endoscopy (VCE) examinations.

ARTIFICIAL INTELLIGENCE IN VIDEO CAPSULE ENDOSCOPY

VCE is an ideal platform for AI utilization and for the development of CNN models for several reasons. First, individual VCE examinations comprise tens of thousands of images, and existing VCE reading software easily creates and maintains a structured image database needed for AI model development. Second, findings on VCE encompass a wide range of pathologic conditions, including luminal bleeding, angioectasias, masses, ulcerations, and many other mucosal alterations. Many of these findings are discrete and are usually annotated during index VCE examinations, which can further simplify AI model development. Third, there is a clinical need for the development of VCE-centered CNN models. Depending on the comfort and expertise of the reader, physician evaluations of VCE examinations can be lengthy. Long reading times and subsequent physician fatigue could be associated with missed findings because many notable lesions are only visible on one or 2 frames. Thus, an AI model that reliably isolates findings to assist readers would be valuable. Finally, VCE is the gold-standard diagnostic tool used for the luminal evaluation of the small bowel, but given its noninvasive nature, the use of VCE is expanding beyond the small bowel. New VCE models provide examinations of the stomach, duodenum, and colon. Furthermore, some capsule models now are capable of pan-endoscopy. Thus, VCE opens up the possibility to noninvasively evaluate epithelial and mucosal lesions dispersed throughout the entire gastrointestinal (GI) tract.[11–19]

In this article, the authors discuss AI models developed for various pathologic processes commonly evaluated on VCE.

TUMOR/POLYP DETECTION

Similar to colonoscopy-based AI models developed for colon polyp detection, researchers have designed VCE-based models to identify protruding lesions of the small bowel and the colon (**Fig. 1**). Different model development techniques can enable autonomous polyp detection from VCE images. For example, researchers have used supervised extraction techniques to allow their model to study and learn color patterns, textures, and shapes from various VCE images. The model then applies what it has learned to images that include polyps and to images that do not. Developers then use the extracted information, separated by classification, to train the model so that it can later distinguish and recognize images containing polyps from normal images in a test data set.[20–22]

A study by Li and colleagues[20] illustrated this concept. In their study, the investigators used a complex schema to train their model using color and shape feature analyses. They developed a complicated algorithm to perform these analyses, as capsule movement through the small bowel naturally results in illumination heterogeneity between frames. This variation in illumination makes color-based analyses quite difficult. The investigators' model used a novel color/shape analytical method that was 94% accurate, 93% specific, and 95% sensitive for detecting polyps.

A

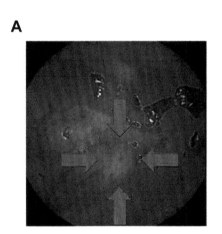

B

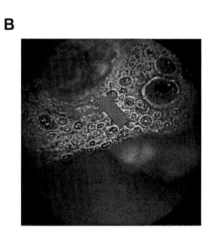

Fig. 1. VCE images of a small bowel polyp (A) and a small bowel mass (B), which are indicated by arrows. (A) One can appreciate the relative subtlety of small bowel polyps, and in this case, the bubbles that help outline the shape of the polyp and assist in identification. (B) The shape and the color of the mass are useful for identification.

CNN models have also been applied to polyp detection. Researchers applying CNNs to VCE studies have used different baseline architectures to develop models tasked with identifying images that contain polyps.[23] In 1 study, researchers used a database of 30,000 VCE images of protruding lesions from 290 patient examinations to develop a CNN model. The CNN model developed from this database was 90% sensitive and 79% specific when tasked with identifying test images containing protruding lesions. Subset analyses evaluating model performance for different lesions demonstrated that the model was 86% sensitive for detecting polyps, 92% sensitive for detecting nodules, 95% sensitive for detecting epithelial-based tumors, 77% sensitive for detecting submucosal lesions, and 94% sensitive for identifying protruding venous structures, such as varices.[24]

Researchers have also developed VCE-based CNNs specifically to identify colonic polyps. This application is intriguing, as a high-performing AI model paired with VCE could potentially serve as an alternative to conventional colonoscopy for colorectal cancer screening. The task of developing a VCE-based CNN to autonomously detect colon polyps is daunting given the broad spectrum of appearance, color, texture, and size of colonic polyps. In addition, relative to the images obtained via newer-generation, high-definition colonoscopes, VCE images may be of poorer quality and are prone to include artifacts (eg, bubbles and fecal matter). Despite that, VCE is a noninvasive, sedationless procedure that could be an attractive alternative to colonoscopy for patients and providers. In order for VCE to be seriously considered as an alternative to colonoscopy, however, an AI system designed to assist in colon polyp detection may be necessary to amplify accuracy. Thus, the development of AI models for colon polyp detection on VCE is now a rapidly growing area of research.

For example, 1 recent study evaluated 255 patients who underwent both a colon capsule endoscopy (CCE) and colonoscopy for the evaluation of colorectal polyps and used that data to generate an AI model. Researchers used a matching algorithm to couple polyps seen on CCE with those detected on colonoscopy. Image features included polyp orientation, polyp location, overall colon cleanliness, polyp size, and polyp morphology. This analysis demonstrated the model was able to perfectly match polyps identified on CCE with those identified on colonoscopy. In addition, the CNN model in this case was 97% sensitive, 93% specific, and 96% accurate for autonomous polyp detection when compared with expert CCE reads.[25]

In another study, by Yuan and Meng,[23] the investigators used a unique deep feature learning method, which they found to be highly accurate for identifying colonic polyps using VCE. Their system used a sparse autoencoder (SAE)-based neural network to generate their model. SAEs are components of deep neural networks that perform unsupervised learning. In this study, SAEs were combined with an "image manifold constraint" system to generate the novel deep learning method. Typically, SAE-based models evaluate and learn features from images individually and do not consider whether images are similar to one another. Conversely, an image manifold constraint system groups similar images together for the purpose of high-level feature learning, which is relevant as consecutive images of a polyp identified on a VCE are likely to have the same valuable, higher-level features that can be used to train an AI system. Thus, the investigators created a "stacked sparse autoencoder with image manifold constraint" system for their analysis. This novel system generated a classification model that was 98% accurate for colon polyp detection. This study also demonstrated that the model developed using this deep feature learning method system had greater accuracy compared with previously studied CNN models designed for the same purpose.

Further evaluation and development of AI models paired with CCE are critical for supporting initiatives for CCE to be considered as an alternative screening tool for colorectal cancer.

GASTROINTESTINAL BLEEDING AND ANGIOECTASIAS

Patients presenting with suspected gastrointestinal bleeding (GIB) can be a diagnostic challenge for clinicians, as potential sources can originate anywhere from the naso-pharynx to the anus. Although many bleeding lesions can be discovered using tradi-tional endoscopic approaches (ie, esophagogastroduodenoscopy [EGD] or colonoscopy), VCE offers many unique benefits compared with these methods. First, VCE allows for direct visualization of regions of the small bowel that are beyond the reach of traditional endoscopy. Second, clinicians can provide capsules to patients quickly on presentation, thus increasing the likelihood that a true culprit lesion will be identified. Finally, newer capsule systems offer important new features, such as a real-time viewer built into the battery pack/recorder, or have been developed based on specific imaging strategies that allow for both pan-endoscopy and region-specific evaluations (ie, upper GI tract capsules vs small bowel capsules vs colon capsules). Thus, there is the potential for nuanced, noninvasive approaches to GIB patients centered on VCE.

Provided that capsules travel several meters in search of bleeding lesions, such as angioectasias (that may only measure a few millimeters in size), methods to narrow the focus of capsule readers to particular video segments are highly desirable. In an attempt to provide a computer-aided diagnosis system for VCE, capsule manufac-turers have worked for years on "suspected blood indicator" (SBI) systems to help cli-nicians localize specific capsule images containing blood within the whole VCE video (**Fig. 2**). SBI software functions work by identifying video frames containing large groups or numbers of red-colored pixels and marking those segments for capsule

A   **B**

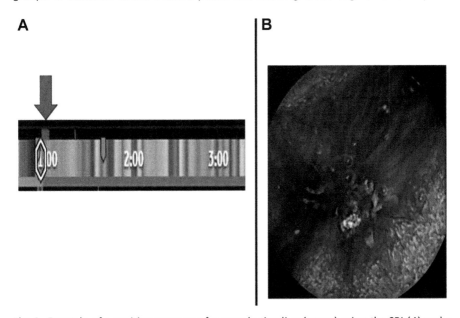

Fig. 2. Example of a positive segment of a capsule timeline (*arrow*) using the SBI (*A*) and a corresponding VCE image from that segment (*B*).

readers. Manufacturers introduced the first SBI used for the detection of potentially bleeding lesions in 2003. The initial evaluation of this technology demonstrated that SBIs are associated with moderate sensitivity and specificity with an overall good negative predictive value.[26–28] A more recent study evaluating an updated version of the SBI demonstrated that the presence of 8 consecutive marked images was associated with 100% sensitivity and 100% specificity for detecting active bleeding, but other studies have suggested that, although SBI markings are highly sensitive for bleeding, they are also associated with low specificity.[29] Furthermore, studies have not shown SBIs to be adequate for identifying lesions that are likely sources of bleeding, such as angioectasias.[30,31]

Clinicians require a method to localize angioectasias more reliably from capsule videos. Angioectasias are the most common source of small bowel bleeding and are responsible for approximately 6% of all cases of GIB.[32] Provided that angioectasias are only visualized over a fraction of the frames of an entire VCE video, and given the difficulty, time, effort, and potential human error involved in reading an entire VCE video, an AI system dedicated to angioectasia identification and localization is attractive to clinicians.[33]

Recent studies have started using newer deep learning approaches to generate models for the task of GI angioectasia identification. A 2018 study by Leenhardt and colleagues[34] used a CNN-based segmentation model developed using still frames from a large, multicenter database of angioectasias obtained during VCE examinations. Of these images, an expert panel identified 600 to be "typical" GI angioectasias. Researchers mixed these images with 600 normal still frame images. They then divided the collection of images into training and test sets and used the training set to develop a CNN model tasked with localizing and identifying angioectasias within a single VCE image. The team assessed CNN model performance using the findings of the expert human panel as a gold standard. The model had high-performance characteristics with a sensitivity of 100%, specificity of 96%, positive predictive value of 96%, and negative predictive value of 100%.

The investigators only briefly discussed one of the most interesting aspects of this study: the difficulties encountered when they initially relied on handcrafted segmentation. Specifically, the investigators described that in their initial approach they used a colorimetric method for training their model, whereby experts identified key features of angioectasias (ie, shape, color, size). They were disappointed, however, with the results of this approach, so the investigators chose to alter course and use a CNN model for feature extraction and training instead of relying on expert-driven feature identification. Without providing specifics, the investigators did note that when using a CNN model their results improved substantially.

Building off the impressive results CNN-based angioectasia detection has demonstrated thus far for, the development and utilization of more advanced CNN models are likely required to further optimize identification accuracy.

CELIAC DISEASE

Celiac disease is an immune condition that results in damage to the small bowel epithelium. The diagnosis of celiac disease is based on a combination of laboratory, endoscopic, and histologic findings. Traditionally, clinicians perform endoscopic evaluation of patients with clinical symptoms or laboratory findings concerning for celiac disease via EGD, but they have considered a role for VCE in the evaluation of celiac disease as well. A previous study of confirmed celiac disease patients demonstrated that VCE was capable of detecting relevant mucosal changes in 85% of patients compared with 80% on EGD.[35] Additional studies have also demonstrated that VCE has greater sensitivity for diagnosing celiac disease than EGD alone.[36,37]

Thus, the potential for image-based AI to assist with the diagnosis of celiac disease using VCE as a platform is promising especially given that researchers have already developed CNN models using EGD images. A previous study demonstrated that an EGD-based CNN algorithm was successful in classifying duodenal mucosa as normal or atrophic and in accurately diagnosing celiac disease.[38]

One of the first studies of AI using a VCE platform used a training data set of 400 VCE images comprising patients with and without celiac disease to train a CNN classification model. Researchers used GoogleNet architecture to generate a CNN model that was 100% sensitive and 100% specific for the evaluation of celiac disease on a test data set. Although these results are impressive, only a small number of patients (11 patients with celiac disease and 10 control patients) were used in the analysis.[39]

More research is needed to better understand the utility of AI models for VCE recognition of celiac disease and its complications. For example, various AI techniques have been proposed for both VCE and endoscopy to enhance images obtained during examination and extract additional information while simultaneously eliminating alterations, including rotation direction, irregular light illumination artifact, and secretions. The application of such techniques for the evaluation of celiac disease may be useful. Specifically, development of systems comprising multiple CNN models used to classify celiac disease and remove undesirable images comprising artifact may be key to the development of an optimal algorithm. Additional areas of study include the development of VCE-based CNN models that can predict clinical outcomes and complications in celiac patients based on image analysis alone.

CROHN DISEASE

Crohn disease (CD) is a chronic inflammatory condition that can affect the entire GI tract, but commonly manifests within the small bowel. Radiologic or endoscopic evaluation of inflammation of the small bowel is key to establishing diagnoses as well as monitoring disease activity for CD patients. The role of VCE in the management of CD is evolving. Historically, computed tomography enterography (CTE) or magnetic resonance enterography (MRE) have been more commonly used tools to evaluate and monitor small bowel inflammation in CD patients. Increasingly, VCE is being used in CD patients and has been shown to have similar diagnostic yields when compared with CTE or MRE (**Fig. 3**).[40] Computer vision techniques similar to those described earlier in this article could further improve yields of VCE in CD patients and allow for new insights into disease characterizations.

Thus far, 1 research group has provided 2 studies evaluating the potential for deep learning algorithms to identify and grade severity of mucosal changes in CD patients. The aim of the first study was to develop a CNN model that could correctly differentiate normal mucosa from ulcerated mucosa in CD patients. The data set in this study comprised 17,640 VCE images extracted from 49 patients (38 with CD and 11 without CD). Researchers annotated images from both groups of patients as having normal mucosa or ulcerated mucosa. Subsequently, they performed 2 experiments, one involving extensive cross-validation to generate a final model and another using per-patient analysis on the training data set. The first experiment demonstrated that the CNN algorithm was 95% to 96% accurate for autonomously detecting ulcerated mucosa and the second experiment demonstrated the per-patient level areas under the receiver operating characteristics ranged from 0.94 to 0.99 for the same task.[41] In the second study from this group, researchers used the same image set with a

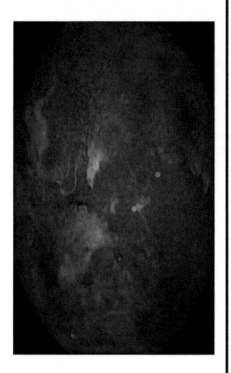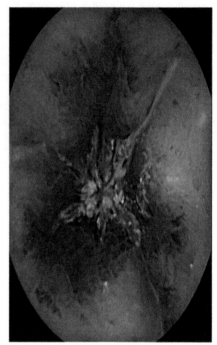

Fig. 3. Side-by-side examples of small bowel CD visualized by VCE.

new aim to train a CNN to accurately grade ulcer severity. In this study, researchers randomly selected 2598 images from the original data set for experts to annotate based on the severity of the mucosal ulceration. They then used a subset of these images to train and test a CNN model. The final model was 91% accurate in distinguishing low-grade ulcerations from severe disease.[42]

Although these studies are impressive, there is much work left to be done in the space. Could, for example, a CNN be trained to differentiate small bowel ulcers identified on VCE by cause (eg, CD, celiac disease, nonsteroidal anti-inflammatory drug induced)? Or, could a CNN be developed to not only evaluate disease activity, but also predict treatment response and eventual need for escalation to biologic therapy or surgery? Additional studies exploring these and other clinical questions could advance the role of VCE-based AI in the diagnosis and management of CD.

SUMMARY

In this section, the authors have reviewed the current state of AI research applied to VCE. Compared with other endoscopic procedures, VCE is well positioned as a focus of AI research going forward. Given the expanding role of VCE in the management of various GI disorders and the massive database of annotated images already available to researchers, it is feasible that VCE will be the endoscopic platform used to establish new AI modeling techniques. In the future, clinicians should expect new VCE-based deep learning models to be developed for colon polyp detection, for providing predictions regarding prognosis of small bowel CD, and for identification of patients afflicted with celiac disease. As AI research centered on VCE becomes more prevalent, clinicians should also anticipate the further establishment of VCE as the key modality for the diagnosis of small bowel diseases and, potentially, the entire GI tract.

DISCLOSURE

Dr P. Sullivan, Dr S. Gupta, and Mr P.D. Powers have no conflict of interest to disclose; Dr N.B. Marya was a consultant for AnX Robotica in the last 2 years.

REFERENCES

1. Baxt WG. Use of an artificial neural network for the diagnosis of myocardial infarction. Ann Intern Med 1991;115(11):843–8.
2. Gulshan V, Peng L, Coram M, et al. Development and validation of a deep learning algorithm for detection of diabetic retinopathy in retinal fundus photographs. JAMA 2016;316(22):2402–10.
3. Karakitsos P, Stergiou EB, Pouliakis A, et al. Potential of the back propagation neural network in the discrimination of benign from malignant gastric cells. Anal Quant Cytol Histol 1996;18(3):245–50.
4. Lucht R, Delorme S, Brix G. Neural network-based segmentation of dynamic MR mammographic images. Magn Reson Imaging 2002;20(2):147–54.
5. Ramesh AN, Kambhampati C, Monson JR, et al. Artificial intelligence in medicine. Ann R Coll Surg Engl 2004;86(5):334–8.
6. Urban G, Tripathi P, Alkayali T, et al. Deep learning localizes and identifies polyps in real time with 96% accuracy in screening colonoscopy. Gastroenterology 2018; 155(4):1069–78.e8.
7. Zachariah R, Samarasena J, Luba D, et al. Prediction of polyp pathology using convolutional neural networks achieves "resect and discard" thresholds. Am J Gastroenterol 2020;115(1):138–44.
8. Le Berre C, Sandborn WJ, Aridhi S, et al. Application of artificial intelligence to gastroenterology and hepatology. Gastroenterology 2020;158(1):76–94 e72.
9. Zhu M, Xu C, Yu J, et al. Differentiation of pancreatic cancer and chronic pancreatitis using computer-aided diagnosis of endoscopic ultrasound (EUS) images: a diagnostic test. PLoS One 2013;8(5):e63820.
10. Wang K, Lu X, Zhou H, et al. Deep learning radiomics of shear wave elastography significantly improved diagnostic performance for assessing liver fibrosis in chronic hepatitis B: a prospective multicentre study. Gut 2019;68(4):729–41.
11. Committee AT, Wang A, Banerjee S, et al. Wireless capsule endoscopy. Gastrointest Endosc 2013;78(6):805–15.
12. Eliakim R, Fireman Z, Gralnek IM, et al. Evaluation of the PillCam Colon capsule in the detection of colonic pathology: results of the first multicenter, prospective, comparative study. Endoscopy 2006;38(10):963–70.
13. Shiotani A, Honda K, Kawakami M, et al. Analysis of small-bowel capsule endoscopy reading by using Quickview mode: training assistants for reading may produce a high diagnostic yield and save time for physicians. J Clin Gastroenterol 2012;46(10):e92–5.

14. Iakovidis DK, Koulaouzidis A. Software for enhanced video capsule endoscopy: challenges for essential progress. Nat Rev Gastroenterol Hepatol 2015;12(3): 172–86.

15. Mustafa BF, Samaan M, Langmead L, et al. Small bowel video capsule endoscopy: an overview. Expert Rev Gastroenterol Hepatol 2013;7(4):323–9.

16. Iddan G, Meron G, Glukhovsky A, et al. Wireless capsule endoscopy. Nature 2000;405(6785):417.

17. MacLeod C, Monaghan E, Banerjee A, et al. Colon capsule endoscopy. Surgeon 2020;18(4):251–6.

18. Yu M. M2A capsule endoscopy. A breakthrough diagnostic tool for small intestine imaging. Gastroenterol Nurs 2002;25(1):24–7.

19. Lee NM, Eisen GM. 10 years of capsule endoscopy: an update. Expert Rev Gastroenterol Hepatol 2010;4(4):503–12.

20. Li B, Meng MQ. Tumor recognition in wireless capsule endoscopy images using textural features and SVM-based feature selection. IEEE Trans Inf Technol Biomed 2012;16(3):323–9.

21. Silva J, Histace A, Romain O, et al. Towards real-time in situ polyp detection in WCE images using a boosting-based approach. Annu Int Conf IEEE Eng Med Biol Soc 2013;2013:5711–4.

22. Charisis VS, Hadjileontiadis LJ, Liatsos CN, et al. Capsule endoscopy image analysis using texture information from various colour models. Comput Methods Programs Biomed 2012;107(1):61–74.

23. Yuan Y, Meng MQ. Deep learning for polyp recognition in wireless capsule endoscopy images. Med Phys 2017;44(4):1379–89.

24. Saito H, Aoki T, Aoyama K, et al. Automatic detection and classification of protruding lesions in wireless capsule endoscopy images based on a deep convolutional neural network. Gastrointest Endosc 2020;92(1):144–51.e1.

25. Blanes-Vidal V, Baatrup G, Nadimi ES. Addressing priority challenges in the detection and assessment of colorectal polyps from capsule endoscopy and colonoscopy in colorectal cancer screening using machine learning. Acta Oncol 2019;58(supp 1):S29–36.

26. Boal Carvalho P, Magalhaes J, Dias DECF, et al. Suspected blood indicator in capsule endoscopy: a valuable tool for gastrointestinal bleeding diagnosis. Arquivos de gastroenterologia 2017;54(1):16–20.

27. Liangpunsakul S, Mays L, Rex DK. Performance of given suspected blood indicator. Am J Gastroenterol 2003;98(12):2676–8.

28. Ghosh T, Fattah SA, Shahnaz C, et al. An automatic bleeding detection scheme in wireless capsule endoscopy based on histogram of an RGB-indexed image. Annu Int Conf IEEE Eng Med Biol Soc 2014;2014:4683–6.

29. Han S, Fahed J, Cave DR. Suspected blood indicator to identify active gastrointestinal bleeding: a prospective validation. Gastroenterol Res 2018;11(2):106–11.

30. D'Halluin PN, Delvaux M, Lapalus MG, et al. Does the "suspected blood indicator" improve the detection of bleeding lesions by capsule endoscopy? Gastrointest Endosc 2005;61(2):243–9.

31. Yung DE, Sykes C, Koulaouzidis A. The validity of suspected blood indicator software in capsule endoscopy: a systematic review and meta-analysis. Expert Rev Gastroenterol Hepatol 2017;11(1):43–51.

32. Foutch PG. Angiodysplasia of the gastrointestinal tract. Am J Gastroenterol 1993; 88(6):807–18.

33. Zheng Y, Hawkins L, Wolff J, et al. Detection of lesions during capsule endoscopy: physician performance is disappointing. Am J Gastroenterol 2012; 107(4):554–60.

34. Leenhardt R, Vasseur P, Li C, et al. A neural network algorithm for detection of GI angiectasia during small-bowel capsule endoscopy. Gastrointest Endosc 2019; 89(1):189–94.

35. Hopper AD, Sidhu R, Hurlstone DP, et al. Capsule endoscopy: an alternative to duodenal biopsy for the recognition of villous atrophy in coeliac disease? Dig Liver Dis 2007;39(2):140–5.

36. Petroniene R, Dubcenco E, Baker JP, et al. Given capsule endoscopy in celiac disease: evaluation of diagnostic accuracy and interobserver agreement. Am J Gastroenterol 2005;100(3):685–94.

37. Rondonotti E, Spada C, Cave D, et al. Video capsule enteroscopy in the diagnosis of celiac disease: a multicenter study. Am J Gastroenterol 2007;102(8): 1624–31.

38. Ciaccio EJ, Bhagat G, Lewis SK, et al. Suggestions for automatic quantitation of endoscopic image analysis to improve detection of small intestinal pathology in celiac disease patients. Comput Biol Med 2015;65:364–8.

39. Zhou T, Han G, Li BN, et al. Quantitative analysis of patients with celiac disease by video capsule endoscopy: a deep learning method. Comput Biol Med 2017; 85:1–6.

40. Yang DH, Keum B, Jeen YT. Capsule endoscopy for crohn's disease: current status of diagnosis and management. Gastroenterol Res Pract 2016;2016:8236367.

41. Klang E, Barash Y, Margalit RY, et al. Deep learning algorithms for automated detection of Crohn's disease ulcers by video capsule endoscopy. Gastrointest Endosc 2020;91(3):606–13.e2.

42. Yiftach B, Liran A, Soffer S, et al. Ulcer severity grading in video-capsule images of Crohn's disease patients: an ordinal neural network solution. Gastrointest Endosc 2020;93(1):187–92.

Novel Clinical Applications and Technical Developments in Video Capsule Endoscopy

Shahrad Hakimian, MD, Mark Hanscom, MD,
David R. Cave, MD, PhD*

KEYWORDS

- Video capsule endoscopy • Small intestine • Innovation • Imaging

KEY POINTS

- Video capsule endoscopy is now being used outside the small bowel in the management of acute gastrointestinal bleeding, including patients with hematemesis and nonhematemesis bleeding and for the diagnosis of colonic neoplasia.
- Novel approaches to imaging beyond white light are being actively investigated for incorporation into capsules to provide additional information at the mucosa level and deeper.
- Technology is rapidly developing for self-propelled capsules that could be deployed for both diagnostic and therapeutic purposes.
- Novel diagnostic approaches are being developed that could be deployed within conventional capsules; these include optical biopsy and tissue biopsy.
- Active investigation is proceeding into therapeutic areas, including drug delivery locally or more generally, and using capsules as therapeutic devices, such as the vibrating capsule in the treatment of constipation.

 Video content accompanies this article at http://www.giendo.theclinics.com/.

INTRODUCTION

Wireless video capsule endoscopy (VCE) first appeared as a clinically useful device in 2001 for imaging the small intestine.[1] Since then, its clinical applications have expanded from examining the small bowel to examining the entire gastrointestinal (GI) tract. The original M_2A device (Given Imaging, Yokneam, Israel) has spawned worldwide interest in the promise of a noninvasive approach to the diagnosis and treatment of intestinal disease. From the early low-resolution images to the current high-definition videos, the entire intestinal tract can now be examined with a very

Department of Medicine, Division of Gastroenterology, University of Massachusetts Medical School, 55 Lake Avenue North, Worcester, MA 01778, USA
* Corresponding author.
E-mail address: david.cave@umassmemorial.org

Gastrointest Endoscopy Clin N Am 31 (2021) 399–412
https://doi.org/10.1016/j.giec.2020.12.011

low miss rate of significant pathologic condition. Going forward, further evolution of this technology will depend considerably on economic issues as well as its acceptance by the medical profession.

The role of VCE in the clinical setting continues to evolve. The original application of VCE was the detection small intestinal bleeding, and it has proven to be effective in that role (see the Daniel L Raines and Douglas G. Adler's article, "The Role of Provocative Testing and Localization of the Video Capsule Endoscope in the Management of Small Intestinal Bleeding," in this issue). There have now been several randomized studies demonstrating VCE has a role in the management of patients with acute GI bleeding. In the case of hematemesis, VCE has been demonstrated to reduce the number of patients requiring admission, and the number of endoscopies required for treatment.[2] In the case of nonhematemesis, VCE has been demonstrated to improve the rate of detection of the site of bleeding compared with patients undergoing standard of care (hazard ratio = 2.7)[3] Earlier investigation improves the likelihood of detecting active bleeding,[4] because most bleeding stops spontaneously, and in 90% of cases, VCE is possible earlier than conventional endoscopy after admission. Ten percent of patients will be too unstable on presentation to tolerate expedited VCE, and this group of patients often requires intensive care unit admission. Following VCE, review of the images can lead to the rapid detection of bleeding using the color bar and suspected blood indicator (SBI) to locate sites of active bleeding. Once located, site-directed endoscopy can then be performed, if needed. The full read of the VCE can be finished at a later time. In comparison, the standard of care, conventional endoscopy, often occurs 12 to 24 hours after admission and can involve a cleaning preparation; in the case of colonoscopy, the cleaning preparation might wash away small amounts of blood that can indicate the source of bleeding. Outside of its role in the detection of active bleeding, VCE can be used for remote diagnosis. The CapsoCam (Intromedic Ltd, Seoul, South Korea) has 4 cameras and stores image data within the capsule itself. This approach is not helpful in acute bleeding but is convenient for gastroenterologists, who do not do frequent VCE and do not need or want a full workstation. The capsule can be swallowed, recovered in a collection kit, and sent to a central reading laboratory with a full report later returned to the referring gastroenterologist.

In addition to the stomach and small bowel, the esophagus has long been considered a potential organ for application of VCE.[5] To date, imaging for esophagitis is the 1 accepted application of VCE in the esophagus. Although there have been attempts with free-floating capsules to image Barrett's esophagus and esophageal varices, VCE has thus far been inferior to conventional endoscopy because of the rapid transit and absence of insufflation. However, newer devices, discussed later in this article, have the potential to remedy the situation. The Navi-Cam capsule (Ankon Technologies Co, Ltd, Wuhan, Shanghai, China) can be released from a tether, after examining the esophagus, for magnetically controlled examination of the stomach.[6] VCE is also of use in the colon, where a colon capsule has been demonstrated to be comparable in diagnostic terms compared with conventional colonoscopy.[7] Even now, despite good evidence that colonoscopy reduces the incidence of colon cancer, many of the general public have been reluctant to undergo this procedure, with participation rates between 50% and 70%. VCE, as a noninvasive alternative, could help improve on this inadequate figure. However, widespread acceptance for this indication faces resistance in endoscopic communities and third-party payers, who are reluctant to replace the safe, but invasive and expensive, fiberoptic video methods in place since the 1970s.

Despite VCE's record of success, there are obstacles to its more complete adoption of VCE. For one, VCE does not have therapeutic capabilities. This absence has proven to be a major stumbling block in its widespread use as a diagnostic tool, as insurance companies would need to (and have been reluctant to) reimburse for both a diagnostic VCE and later a therapeutic colonoscopy in up to 50% of patients. Second, cost remains a concern. Capsules are semiconductor devices that are now being produced in large quantities by multiple manufacturers. Nevertheless, there has been little to no cost reduction, despite this being the case with personal computers and similar semiconductor-based devices. Third, linear localization also remains a problem. Capsule endoscopists use a time-based approach to measure how far the capsule has traveled along the GI tract. To do this, the small intestine is first divided into tertiles or quartiles, based on the timestamp of the pylorus and ileocecal valve. Then, best estimates are made to predict the location of the lesion with respect to these 2 fixed points. This approach has significant limitations, particularly if the capsule is retained or otherwise held up at a point, or if there is incomplete transit. Transient retentions in these situations can lead to misleading interpretations of the exact location of the lesion. More accurate information on how far the capsule has traveled would be a great asset to the therapeutic endoscopist or surgeon.

Nevertheless, the future of VCE is bright, with several advancements in imaging, locomotion, diagnostic, and therapeutic capabilities promising to further revolutionize the field, and even more advancements on the horizon. Localization in 3 dimensions has been solved using built-in software using radiofrequency (RF) and is now commercially available. Localization by measuring changes in magnetic field is evolving and potentially offers localization in the colon down into the millimeter range. Localization is further aided by the introduction of a complementary device, the powered spiral enteroscope,[8] which has the potential to be passed through the mouth all the way to the ileocecal valve for therapeutic purposes.

The rapidly developing field of artificial intelligence (AI) is certain to play a significant role, as it could relieve the capsule operator of the tedium of reviewing of one or more video streams from the capsule camera. The point at which optical biopsy (histology assessed by AI) can be performed with a high degree of reliability is approaching. Optical biopsy could greatly diminish the role of therapeutics at the time of primary colonoscopy, as only 10% of the population has advanced adenomas during index colonoscopy, and thus would spare 90% of patients the need for therapeutic colonoscopy. Those patients with small adenomas can then be safely left to subsequent surveillance colonoscopy 5 to 7 years after initial examination. Even now, repeat screening or surveillance with a low need for therapeutic intervention could be performed with the colon capsule. The ability to localize polyps in the colon with a high degree of accuracy using these new technologies could allow for serial observations that a specific polyp has either remained the same or grown in a suspicious manner.

Finally, the COVID-19 epidemic has provided an opportunity for the further use of VCE in acute GI bleeding. The authors are in the process of completing a trial comparing standard-of-care versus capsule-first endoscopy to examine how VCE might reduce the number of conventional procedures needed. Compared with conventional endoscopy, VCE produces no significant aerosols during ingestion and still provides excellent imaging of the GI tract. VCE-first algorithms might allow for minimizing the use of personal protective equipment and limitation of viral exposure for personnel. Preliminary data suggest such an approach can reduce the number of procedures needed by 54% with similar outcomes in terms of safety and rebleeding in patients with both hematemesis and nonhematemesis presenting GI bleeding.

ADVANCEMENTS IN IMAGING

Since its inception, VCE has benefited from significant technological improvements in image enhancement and capture. Included in these improvements are wider angles of view, more sophisticated camera lenses, automated control of light exposure, increased battery capacity, and advanced AI.

Improvements in camera technologies and light control have led to better visualization of GI mucosa. Different variations of cameras and light conditions have been evaluated to allow for better visualization and increasing diagnostic yield of capsule endoscopes under various conditions. Although most current standard capsule endoscopes have only 1 recording camera, 2- and 4-camera capsules have now been developed. Some studies show that the diagnostic yield can be higher with the use of more than 1 camera,[9] perhaps because as the capsule tumbles throughout the GI tract fewer lesions can be masked under mucosal folds based on the angle of view. However, an increase in the number of recording cameras also equates to an increase in battery usage, data recording, and length of viewing time, which remains a sizable barrier to the implementation.

In addition to improved cameras, improved methods of imaging have also been introduced. White-light endoscopy (WLE) has been the traditional approach used to evaluate lesions in both video capsule and tethered endoscopes. However, although WLE allows for great visualization of mucosal surfaces (and even greater now with high-definition cameras), non–white-light endoscopy (NWLE) can enable visualization of deeper mucosal layers and allow for better diagnoses of certain luminal masses. Different variations of NWLE have been evaluated. For example, flexible spectral imaging color enhancement (FICE) is a digital algorithm that takes white-light images, emphasizes specific wavelengths of light in the red, green, and blue spectrums, and produces a final amalgamation of an image that is meant to delineate luminal lesions.[10] Although FICE is thought to improve delineation of luminal ulcers and angioectasias compared with WLE, 1 meta-analysis suggests this benefit is derived from FICE 1 mode alone, and FICE 2 and FICE 3 were without benefit.[11] Narrowband imaging (NBI) is another method of imaging that has been proposed for better visualization of mucosal vessels. Although NBI has not yet made its way into commercial capsule endoscopes, designs and engineering constructs have been developed[12] for its integration into the capsule endoscope in the future. One form of this technology, so-called blue-light endoscopy, has been evaluated in the detection of GI lesions with controversial results. Blue-light endoscopy uses a color coefficient shift of light in the short wavelength range (490–430 nm) superimposed onto white light. In 1 trial comparing the use of blue-light endoscopy in the detection of small intestinal lesions, it was found to have no benefit over WLE alone.[13]

In addition to improvements to old technologies in cameras and light imaging, new methods have been developed to improve submucosal imaging. Microultrasound and thermometric capsule endoscopy are being developed to provide subsurface images of the small bowel using frequency $\geq$30 MHz, which can complement optical information provided by VCE.[14] The ultrasonic frequency in these devices compares with traditional endoscopic ultrasounds that function in the range of 12 to 20 MHz. Sonocap, for example, is one such device that contains 4 single-element spherically focused microultrasound transducers that allow for visualization of different layers of the bowel wall. Fluorescent-enhanced VCE is another technology that might find its way into capsule endoscopy in the near future. With the current technology, the distinction between active GI bleeding or recent bleeding with distal passage can be difficult, as in both cases the blood appears red. In fluorescent-enhanced VCE, fluorescent dye can be first injected and then detected via special sensors on the capsule endoscope, mimicking (and, perhaps with optimization, replacing) a nuclear medicine scan. AI with convoluted neural networks is another area in which VCE seems destined to see significant involvement. In current, commercially available VCE systems, the SBI and quick view components allow for rapid identification of red pixels to aid in the detection of bleeding. Unfortunately, the SBI has a relatively low specificity for active small intestinal bleeding. However, 8 contiguous SBI markers have been reported to have strong sensitivity and specificity for active bleeding.[15] In addition, algorithms have been developed to reduce the number of duplicate images and hence reduce the reading time of the capsule data. In the future, AI may assist in the identification of lesions and more accurate localization of the capsule endoscope within the whole GI tract.

Besides technologic advancements in the video capsule itself, the real-time viewer, a feature offered in the most recent editions of VCE recording modules, allows visualization of the capsule recording in real time, allowing several advantages. For example, the real-time viewer can be used to detect the presence of blood/active bleeding in the stomach within a few seconds of capsule ingestion, enabling capsule endoscopy as a powerful screening tool for source-directed endoscopic evaluation. This same technology can be used to detect gastric passage into the duodenum and aid in the decision to use promotility agents to help evacuation in select cases. Finally, the recorder can be used to determine cecal entry and help with shortening the recording time. The future generations of recording modules could benefit from added features, allowing real-time upload of the images to a server for removal of real-time viewing, reduced image download time, cloud storage to allow for remote reading, and educational purposes and consultation.

ADVANCEMENTS IN LOCOMOTION

One of the current major limitations of VCE is its lack of maneuverability. Current applications of VCE thus depend on gravitational and peristaltic forces to transport the capsule forward, which can result in wide variations in transit time between GI segments, limited evaluation of segments with large surface areas, and missed lesions.[16] In response, considerable interest and resources have been devoted to developing new methods for capsule locomotion[17–19] (**Table 1**). Precision navigation promises to position VCE as a leading tool in the safe, noninvasive investigation of a multitude of GI conditions. To date, there have been 2 main strategies for improving locomotion

Table 1
Select advancements in locomotion of endoscopic capsules

Reference, Year	Locomotion	Actuation	Development Stage
Quirini et al,[21] 2008	Internal	Legs	Porcine in vivo
Kim et al,[22] 2010	Internal	Paddling	Porcine in vivo
Kim et al,[24] 2005	Internal	Inchworm	In vitro
De Falco et al,[27] 2014	Internal	Propeller	Ex vivo
Lien et al,[35] 2014	External	Handheld magnet	Ex vivo
Keller et al,[38] 2011	External	Handheld magnet	Human in vivo
Ching et al,[6] 2019	External	Handheld magnet	Human in vivo
Jiang et al,[45] 2020	External	Remote controlled	Human in vivo

in VCE. The first, internal locomotion, involves embedding a miniature actuator on board the capsule to effect locomotion. The second, external locomotion, also referred to as magnet-controlled capsule endoscopy (MCE), involves using magnets to orient and steer the capsule through at least part of the GI tract.

Internal locomotion comprises several different devices using various methods of mechanical actuation.[17–20] Advancements in internal locomotion have been limited by technological constraints, namely, the need to incorporate actuators, other mechanical components, and batteries, into a device small enough to be comfortably swallowed. Nevertheless, several devices have been tested in in vitro and ex vivo models, although clinical models are lacking. These devices have used methods of actuation, including leg-based, paddle-based, earthworm-based, and propeller-based locomotion. The leg-based model consists of an endoscopic capsule with 8 propelling electromechanical legs. The device has been tested in both ex vivo and porcine models, demonstrating success in backward and vertical movement at a speed of 6 cm per minute.[21] Similarly, the paddling-based model, which uses multiple legs that move from front to back to propel the capsule forward, has also demonstrated success in porcine models.[22,23] On the other hand, earthworm-based techniques are meant to mimic the inching movement of an earthworm and consist of shape memory alloy wires that elongate and retract and "clampers" that hook into the GI mucosa and pull the capsule forward by an anchor-and-pull effect.[24,25] Finally, propeller-based models have been among the best-studied internal locomotion devices. Tortora and colleagues[26] developed a 30 × 15-mm capsule containing a wireless microcontroller, a battery, and 4 motors that rotate propellers on the rear of the capsule. The capsule is controlled using a joystick to navigate the gastric mucosa for up to 30 minutes. De Falco and colleagues[27] developed a similar, slightly larger capsule that also incorporates a camera module and can be navigated for up to 13 minutes by looking at a video streaming platform. Similar self-propelling capsule endoscopes have demonstrated success in navigation, object identification, and image acquisition in animal models.[28] Other experimental approaches based on mechanical actuation have included swimming tails, propulsive flaps, and tethered propulsion systems that use water jets to orient the capsule within the stomach.[29–31] Overall, interest in internal locomotion has waned because of the significant technological hurdles, including the need for large power supplies, increased capsule size to house the various components, and the need for safe interaction between mechanical appendages and the GI mucosa. Although improvements in energy storage may ameliorate some of these concerns, for now, the focus has shifted to favor external locomotion.[18]

External locomotion, or MCE, uses the interaction between capsules containing magnetic components and external magnetic fields to alter capsule orientation and direct movement. Compared with internal locomotion, external locomotion has been favored for its technological and engineering advantages and has been better studied in clinical settings.[19,20] The 2 main methods of navigation in MCE are manipulation through handheld magnets and manipulation through robot-guided magnets.[18,19] The former uses human controllers to manually hold magnets outside the patient's torso, whereas the latter uses robotic components (such as a mechanical C-arm) to stabilize external magnets that are then directed remotely by a human controller, often at a nearby or even remote workstation. The first devices to use MCE were introduced by Carpi and colleagues[32] and based on techniques used to steer interventional cardiovascular devices.[33] Carpi's system used elastic shells mixed with magnetic particles that were applied over endoscopic capsules and controlled with external magnetic fields. Since then, progress has accelerated. Valdastri and colleagues[34] developed a capsule that incorporated intracapsular moveable magnets with internal actuation to achieve fine camera control. The camera could thus be rotated and positioned to obtain 360° views of the gastric lumen. Lien and colleagues[35] later introduced the first handheld external controller, allowing the endoscopist to remotely control both the movement of the endoscopic capsule and the angle of the camera module. Similar devices have been tested in humans with promising results. Swain and colleagues[36] demonstrated ease of use of MCE in the stomach and esophagus of healthy volunteers. Likewise, Keller and colleagues[37] demonstrated MCE to be safe and feasible in the evaluation of the esophagus and gastric lumen, with greater than 75% of the gastric mucosa able to be assessed.[38] In 1 trial of 26 volunteers, MCE could be manipulated into the correct position 88% of the time and visualized important anatomic landmarks in 92% to 100% of cases.[23,39] Difficulties were encountered near the esophagogastric junction, where peristaltic forces could overpower the magnetic hold. Currently, there is at least 1 well-studied handheld MCE system being tested in clinical use with the MiroCam. The MiroCam Navi (Intromedic Ltd) consists of a capsule endoscope, an external handheld magnet, a data recorder, an associated workstation for video download, and a tablet that allows for live viewing through a wireless connection. The capsule has an estimated 11-hour battery life.[6] Procedure preparation includes drinking a polyethylene glycol solution the night before the examination in order to clean the gastric lumen, followed by 1 L of water on the morning of examination to distend the stomach and provide a medium for capsule manipulation. The handheld magnet, in combination with patient positional changes, is used to carry the capsule to new positions in the gastric lumen to obtain a full view of the mucosa. In comparative studies, the MiroCam has also shown promising results. Ching and colleagues[6] compared MCE versus conventional esophagogastroduodenoscopy (EGD) in patients with iron-deficiency anemia and found that the MiroCam was better tolerated than EGD and detected more pathologic findings (113 vs 52; $P<.001$).

Robot-guided MCE replaces the human controller with a robotic one, eliminating the unstable movements by hand and hence improving procedural precision.[18] Ciuti and colleagues[40] first demonstrated as much in a comparative trial between robot-guided and handheld control, in which robot-guided control both decreased procedure time (201 seconds vs 423 seconds) and increased the number of intraprocedural targets reached (87% vs 37%). Robot-guided MCE has been well studied in clinical use through use of the NaviCam system. The NaviCam system consists of a capsule endoscope, a guidance magnet robot, a data recorder, and a computer workstation. The capsule measures 26.88×11.6 mm in size, with an estimated battery life of 8 hours, and contains a permanent magnet inside its dome. The endoscopist uses joystick controls to manipulate a robotic C-arm across 2 rotational and 3 translational degrees of freedom, in turn manipulating the direction of the magnetic capsule. The optimal gastric preparation involves ingesting water with simethicone before the examination, which improves detection of findings (67.5%) compared with water alone (52.5%) and water with pronase (53.8%).[41] Gastric cleanliness can also be improved with sequential position changes after simethicone ingestion, which reduces the gastric examination time but not the detection rate of positive findings.[42] The best-studied protocol involves a combination of 5 position changes (supine, left lateral, knee-chest, right lateral, and sitting) to optimize gastric mucosa visualization.[43] In initial studies using the NaviCam in human volunteers, the NaviCam demonstrated good maneuverability, with complete visualization of the gastric cardia, fundus, body, angularis, antrum, and pylorus in 82.4%, 85.3%, 100%, 100%, 100%, and 100% of cases, respectively. The average examination time was 43.8 minutes, and no serious adverse events were reported[44] (Videos 1–3). Similar findings have since been reproduced outside of China, including in Europe. Since then, Ankon has come out with a second-generation MCE that improves upon its predecessor's procedural time, image quality, and maneuverability.[45] To date, there have been several comparative studies between MCE using the NaviCam and conventional endoscopy. Zou and colleagues[46] compared MCE with EGD in 68 patients and found positive agreement in 96% of cases and negative agreement in 77.8% of cases, with a kappa of 0.765. Qian and colleagues[47] found that MCE could detect superficial gastric neoplasia in 10 patients planned for endoscopic submucosal dissection (ESD) with per-patient and per-lesion sensitivities of 100% and 91.7%, respectively. In a large, multicenter, blinded trial, 350 patients with upper abdominal complaints underwent MCE followed by EGD within 2 hours. MCE detected gastric focal lesions with a sensitivity, specificity, positive predictive value, and negative predictive value of 90.4%, 94.7%, 87.9%, and 95.9%, respectively. No lesions of significance (such as tumors or large ulcers) were missed during MCE, and just 5 patients (1.4%) reported adverse events.[48] In another large, observational cohort study, 3182 patients underwent gastric cancer screening using MCE. MCE proved to be safe and feasible as a screening method, detecting 7 total cases of gastric cancer.[35] The mean examination time was 14 minutes. The esophagus has also been independently evaluated using a modified MCE with a detachable string. Detachable string MCE (DS-MCE) was completed with success in all 25 patients studied without adverse events.[49,50] The examination achieved technical success in 100% of cases with no cases of string damage or capsule loss. Compared with EGD, DS-MCE was able to diagnosis varices with a sensitivity of 100% and was able to appropriately grade varices and reflux esophagitis with accuracies of 66.7% and 100%, respectively.[49]

ADVANCEMENTS IN DIAGNOSTICS

Despite the widespread interest in VCE for its ease of use, patient comfort, and noninvasive access to difficult-to-reach areas of the GI tract, its lack of diagnostic and therapeutic capabilities has limited its wider role in clinical practice. Advances in the imaging and locomotion capabilities of VCE have since allowed for stepwise advances in its diagnostic and therapeutic potential, with some estimations that VCE will become the main method of both diagnostic and therapeutic endoscopic procedures within the next 15 years.[51]

The diagnostic advancements in VCE comprise 2 major techniques: optical biopsy and tissue biopsy. Optical biopsy refers to the technique of obtaining a diagnosis without tissue acquisition. Optical biopsy has been tested in several settings, including in the detection of microscopic malignancy, the detection of Barrett's esophagus, and the detection of adenomatous polyps.[52,53] The Compact Photonic Explorer (CPE) is one such device, which has been created and tested in the detection of malignancy. The CPE is a small (5 mm), wireless, spectroscopic-based device that can be manipulated using remote-controlled radio signals and that contains a suite of imaging and biosensing technologies that can detect disease and monitor physiologic functions. In the future, the creators anticipate expanding its capabilities into tissue removal and repair.[52,54] Optical biopsy has also been used with success in patients with Barrett's esophagus. Seibel and colleagues[55] developed a tethered capsule endoscope consisting of a 6.4-mm capsule attached to a tether. The capsule contains a fiberoptic laser scanner that video records high-resolution, wide-field color images as the capsule is retracted after an initial swallow. In a trial of 13 human subjects, distinct differences were seen in the images between patients with Barrett's esophagus and healthy volunteers. The mean procedural time lasted 6 minutes, 18 seconds, and there were no complications.[53,56] A similar technique using string VCE has been used in the diagnosis of esophageal varices. String VCE carried out using the PillCam device (Pill-Cam SB; Given Imaging Ltd) consisted of a plastic sleeve placed over the capsule and tethered to strings. The device was tested in 100 patients and found to have a sensitivity and specificity of clinically significant varices of 82.1 and 90.2 with a kappa of 0.73 compared with varices. Seventy-one percent of patients indicated they preferred VCE over EGD, and no complications were recorded.[57] One slight variation of traditional optical biopsy is bio-chromoendoscopy, in which VCE is modified with probe-based imaging technology in order to detect specific wavelengths of light (so-called molecular beacons) emitted by malignant and premalignant GI lesions. The technique involves injection of a synthetic probe, or "molecular beacon," that remains undetectable in tissue until it is cleaved and activated by local enzymes. Once cleaved, the probe then emits near-infrared fluorescence (NIRF) that can be detected during VCE. Using certain probes that are tailored to be activated by specific enzymes that are upregulated in neoplastic lesions, VCE can thus be used to distinguish neoplastic lesions from normal tissue. Zhang and colleagues[58] have since published a proof-of-principle trial, in which NIRF-integrated VCE was able to detect signal from adenomatous polyps, without overlap among lymphoid polyps, hyperplastic polyps, acute inflammation, or chronic inflammation. Tissue biopsy, on the other hand, refers to the formal acquisition of actual tissue to make a diagnosis. One of the oldest methods of tissue acquisition involved the original Crosby capsule, which used a tethered capsule under fluoroscopic guidance and a Seldinger wire to obtain jejunal biopsies.[59] Newer devices developed to obtain tissue biopsies include a spring-loaded device similar to the Crosby capsule, a device using microspikes with protruding barbs and Microelectromechanical systems (MEMS) technology, and a device using a rotational tissue-cutting razor.[51,54,59] The latter rotational device uses a rotational tissue cutting razor with a torsion spring and has been tested in both a cow and rabbit intestine model with the successful collection of 1-mm samples of tissue.[60] There are now several major multidisciplinary efforts leading the front in advancing capsule technologies. The VECTOR (versatile endoscopic capsule for gastrointestinal tumor recognition and therapy) project is one such effort supported by the European Union with the goal of developing a "miniature robotic pill for advanced diagnostics and therapy in the human gastrointestinal tract."

ADVANCEMENTS IN THERAPEUTICS

In addition to diagnostic capabilities, therapeutic capabilities in VCE have expanded with improvements in imaging and machine learning. There are now multiple devices designed for controlled drug delivery throughout the GI tract.[42] The high-frequency capsule (Battelle-Institute V, Frankfurt am Main, Germany) was developed in the 1980s. It uses RF pulse to generate a current, heating a filament until it melts and releases a needle, which then pierces a balloon to release its contents. Limitations of the high-frequency capsule include the need for x-ray fluoroscopy (and the associated radiation) to track the capsule location, and technical difficulties with filling the balloon.[61] The Gastro Target telemetric capsule (Gastro Target Corp, Tonawanda, NY, USA) also uses an external RF pulse. The RF pulse triggers a needle release, which pierces a balloon, allowing separate chemicals to mix and produce carbon dioxide, which in turn increases pressure and drives a piston pushing out the contents. Limitations include the need to use a dummy capsule 3 days before dosing to determine location. A different capsule, the Telemetric capsule (INSERM U61, Strasbourg Cedex, France), is activated by an external magnet, which releases a compressed spring that allows the drug reservoir to empty. Limitations include prolonged stomach retention because of the size of the device as well as limited battery power and technical difficulties with particulate delivery.[61] Developments in controlled drug delivery have been spurred by the growth in new drugs with complicated pharmaceutical properties and the desire for companies to collect absorption data in a noninvasive manner. Two recent additions to the arsenal include the Intellisite capsule (Innovative Devices, Raleigh, NC, USA) and the Enterion Capsule (Phaeton Research, Nottingham, UK). Both were designed to deliver a wide range of drug formulations (solution, powder, granulate) into various regions of the gut. The latter has been studied in human subjects, with active dispersion of the drug and no serious adverse events.[62] The iPill (Philips Research, Eindhoven, The Netherlands) is a prototype capsule that measures 11 × 26 mm in size, and includes an RF wireless transceiver, internal pump, and microprocessor to allow it to deliver drug in a burst, progressive release, or multilocation dosing. It is being evaluated in patients with Crohn disease and colon cancer.[54]

The diagnostic and therapeutic possibilities of wireless technologies have also been studied in the subfield of neuro-gastroenterology and motility. For example, the Bion, a remote, battery-powered microstimulator designed to be implanted through a minimally invasive procedure, can raise the pressure in the lower esophageal sphincter (LES).[63] The 3.3 × 28-mm microstimulator can be implanted into the LES and increases pressure in a dose-dependent manner up to 3 times higher than baseline as demonstrated in a canine model, offering promise in the treatment of gastroesophageal reflux disease.[64] VCE has also been used to diagnose intestinal motor disorders.[65] For example, in a comparison between 36 subjects with severe intestinal motor disorders and 50 healthy subjects, VCE in combination with machine learning was able to identify patients with intestinal motor disorders based on contractile activity, static sequences, and turbid intestinal content. Endoluminal analysis with computer vision offers promise as a reliable, noninvasive means of diagnosing motility disorders, which has up to this point required specialized technologies at centers of expertise.[65]

SUMMARY

VCE has become the gold standard for diagnosing small intestinal disease. Interest in this noninvasive technology has grown to encompass the entire GI tract. Potential applications for use in the entire GI tract are entering the realms of clinical reality. These applications include the use of AI, self-propelled capsules, novel diagnostic imaging, drug delivery, and many others. This technology is here to stay and is only limited by our imagination.

DISCLOSURE

S. Hakimian, None. M. Hanscom, None. D.R. Cave in receipt of research grant support from Medtronic, Ireland and Olympus, Japan.

SUPPLEMENTARY DATA

Supplementary video related to this article can be found at https://doi.org/10.1016/j.giec.2020.12.011.

CLINIC CARE POINTS

- The VCE technology is rapidly changing and further advancements are enabling evaluation of various upper and lower GI conditions including but not limited to diagnostic evaluation of upper GI bleeding and colon cancer screening.
- Advances in locomotion such as use of magnetic capsules, new imaging techniques, and new capabilities such as drug delivery and biopsy sampling are likely to change the future of capsule endoscopy and enable more widespread use within and beyond the small bowel.

REFERENCES

1. Lewis BS, Swain P. Capsule endoscopy in the evaluation of patients with suspected small intestinal bleeding: results of a pilot study. Gastrointest Endosc 2002;56(3):349–53.
2. Gralnek IM, Ching JY, Maza I, et al. Capsule endoscopy in acute upper gastrointestinal hemorrhage: a prospective cohort study. Endoscopy 2013;45(1):12–9.
3. Marya NB, Jawaid S, Foley A, et al. A randomized controlled trial comparing efficacy of early video capsule endoscopy with standard of care in the approach to nonhematemesis GI bleeding (with videos). Gastrointest Endosc 2019;89(1):33–43 e34.
4. Singh A, Marshall C, Chaudhuri B, et al. Timing of video capsule endoscopy relative to overt obscure GI bleeding: implications from a retrospective study. Gastrointest Endosc 2013;77(5):761–6.
5. Park J, Cho YK, Kim JH. Current and future use of esophageal capsule endoscopy. Clin Endosc 2018;51(4):317–22.
6. Ching H-L, Hale MF, Kurien M, et al. Diagnostic yield of magnetically assisted capsule endoscopy versus gastroscopy in recurrent and refractory iron deficiency anemia. Endoscopy 2019;51(5):409–18.
7. Spada C, Pasha SF, Gross SA, et al. Accuracy of first- and second-generation colon capsules in endoscopic detection of colorectal polyps: a systematic review and meta-analysis. Clin Gastroenterol Hepatol 2016;14(11):1533–1543 e1538.
8. Beyna T, Arvanitakis M, Schneider M, et al. Motorised spiral enteroscopy: first prospective clinical feasibility study. Gut 2020. https://doi.org/10.1136/gutjnl-2019-319908.
9. Triantafyllou K, Papanikolaou IS, Papaxoinis K, et al. Two cameras detect more lesions in the small-bowel than one. World J Gastroenterol 2011;17(11):1462–7.
10. Imagawa H, Oka S, Tanaka S, et al. Improved detectability of small-bowel lesions via capsule endoscopy with computed virtual chromoendoscopy: a pilot study. Scand J Gastroenterol 2011;46(9):1133–7.
11. Yung DE, Boal Carvalho P, Giannakou A, et al. Clinical validity of flexible spectral imaging color enhancement (FICE) in small-bowel capsule endoscopy: a systematic review and meta-analysis. Endoscopy 2017;49(3):258–69.
12. Lan-Rong D, Yin-Yi W. A wireless narrowband imaging chip for capsule endoscope. IEEE Trans Biomed circuits Syst 2010;4(6):462–8.
13. Koulaouzidis A, Douglas S, Plevris JN. Blue mode does not offer any benefit over white light when calculating Lewis score in small-bowel capsule endoscopy. World J Gastrointest Endosc 2012;4(2):33–7.
14. Qiu Y, Huang Y, Zhang Z, et al. Ultrasound capsule endoscopy with a mechanically scanning micro-ultrasound: a porcine study. Ultrasound Med Biol 2020;46(3):796–804.

15. Han S, Fahed J, Cave DR. Suspected blood indicator to identify active gastrointestinal bleeding: a prospective validation. Gastroenterology Res 2018;11(2): 106–11.

16. Keller J, Fibbe C, Rosien U, et al. Recent advances in capsule endoscopy: development of maneuverable capsules. Expert Rev Gastroenterol Hepatol 2012;6(5): 561–6.

17. Kwack WG, Lim YJ. Current status and research into overcoming limitations of capsule endoscopy. Clin Endosc 2016;49(1):8–15.

18. Slawinski PR, Obstein KL, Valdastri P. Capsule endoscopy of the future: what's on the horizon? World J Gastroenterol 2015;21(37):10528–41.

19. Ciuti G, Caliò R, Camboni D, et al. Frontiers of robotic endoscopic capsules: a review. J Microbio Robot 2016;11(1):1–18.

20. Nam S-J, Lee HS, Lim YJ. Evaluation of gastric disease with capsule endoscopy. Clin Endosc 2018;51(4):323–8.

21. Quirini M, Menciassi A, Scapellato S, et al. Feasibility proof of a legged locomotion capsule for the GI tract. Gastrointest Endosc 2008;67(7):1153–8.

22. Kim HM, Yang S, Kim J, et al. Active locomotion of a paddling-based capsule endoscope in an in vitro and in vivo experiment (with videos). Gastrointest Endosc 2010;72(2):381–7.

23. Yang S, Park K, Kim J, et al. Autonomous locomotion of capsule endoscope in gastrointestinal tract. Conf Proc IEEE Eng Med Biol Soc 2011;2011:6659–63.

24. Kim B, Kim B, Lee S, et al. Design and fabrication of a locomotive mechanism for capsule-type endoscopes using shape memory alloys (SMAs). IEEE ASME Trans Mechatron 2005;10(1):77–86.

25. Kim B, Kim Byungkyu, Park Sukho, et al. "An earthworm-like locomotive mechanism for capsule endoscopes," 2005. Edmonton, Alta: IEEE/RSJ International Conference on Intelligent Robots and Systems; 2005. p. 2997–3002.

26. Tortora G, Valdastri P, Susilo E, et al. Propeller-based wireless device for active capsular endoscopy in the gastric district. Minim Invasive Ther Allied Technol 2009;18(5):280–90.

27. De Falco I, Tortora G, Dario P, et al. An integrated system for wireless capsule endoscopy in a liquid-distended stomach. IEEE Trans Biomed Eng 2014;61(3): 794–804.

28. Morita E, Ohtsuka N, Shindo Y, et al. In vivo trial of a driving system for a self-propelling capsule endoscope using a magnetic field (with video). Gastrointest Endosc 2010;72(4):836–40.

29. Kósa G, Jakab P, Székely G, et al. MRI driven magnetic microswimmers. Biomed Microdevices 2012;14(1):165–78.

30. Valdastri P, Sinibaldi S, Caccavaro G. A novel magnetic actuation system for miniature swimming robots 2011;27(1):769–79.

31. Caprara R, Obstein KL, Scozzarro G, et al. A platform for gastric cancer screening in low- and middle-income countries. IEEE Trans Biomed Eng 2015; 62(5):1324–32.

32. Carpi F, Galbiati S, Carpi A. Controlled navigation of endoscopic capsules: concept and preliminary experimental investigations. IEEE Trans Biomed Eng 2007;54(11):2028–36.

33. Carpi F, Pappone C. Magnetic maneuvering of endoscopic capsules by means of a robotic navigation system. IEEE Trans Biomed Eng 2009;56(5):1482–90.

34. Valdastri P, Quaglia C, Buselli E, et al. A magnetic internal mechanism for precise orientation of the camera in wireless endoluminal applications. Endoscopy 2010; 42(6):481–6.

35. Lien G-S, Liu C-W, Jiang J-A, et al. Magnetic control system targeted for capsule endoscopic operations in the stomach–design, fabrication, and in vitro and ex vivo evaluations. IEEE Trans Biomed Eng 2012;59(7):2068–79.
36. Swain P, Toor A, Volke F, et al. Remote magnetic manipulation of a wireless capsule endoscope in the esophagus and stomach of humans (with videos). Gastrointest Endosc 2010;71(7):1290–3.
37. Keller J, Fibbe C, Volke F, et al. Remote magnetic control of a wireless capsule endoscope in the esophagus is safe and feasible: results of a randomized, clinical trial in healthy volunteers. Gastrointest Endosc 2010;72(5):941–6.
38. Keller J, Fibbe C, Volke F, et al. Inspection of the human stomach using remote-controlled capsule endoscopy: a feasibility study in healthy volunteers (with videos). Gastrointest Endosc 2011;73(1):22–8.
39. Rahman I, Pioche M, Shim CS, et al. Magnetic-assisted capsule endoscopy in the upper GI tract by using a novel navigation system (with video). Gastrointest Endosc 2016;83(5):889–95.e881.
40. Ciuti G, Donlin R, Valdastri P, et al. Robotic versus manual control in magnetic steering of an endoscopic capsule. Endoscopy 2010;42(2):148–52.
41. Zhu S-G, Qian Y-Y, Tang X-Y, et al. Gastric preparation for magnetically controlled capsule endoscopy: a prospective, randomized single-blinded controlled trial. Dig Liver Dis 2018;50(1):42–7.
42. Wang Y-C, Pan J, Jiang X, et al. Repetitive position change improves gastric cleanliness for magnetically controlled capsule gastroscopy. Dig Dis Sci 2019;64(5):1297–304.
43. Qian Y, Wu S, Wang Q, et al. Combination of five body positions can effectively improve the rate of gastric mucosa's complete visualization by applying magnetic-guided capsule endoscopy. Gastroenterol Res Pract 2016;2016:6471945.
44. Liao Z, Duan X-D, Xin L, et al. Feasibility and safety of magnetic-controlled capsule endoscopy system in examination of human stomach: a pilot study in healthy volunteers. J Interv Gastroenterol 2012;2(4):155–60.
45. Jiang B, Qian Y-Y, Pan J, et al. Second-generation magnetically controlled capsule gastroscopy with improved image resolution and frame rate: a randomized controlled clinical trial (with video). Gastrointest Endosc 2020;91(6):1379–87.
46. Zou W-B, Hou X-H, Xin L, et al. Magnetic-controlled capsule endoscopy vs. gastroscopy for gastric diseases: a two-center self-controlled comparative trial. Endoscopy 2015;47(6):525–8.
47. Qian Y-Y, Zhu S-G, Hou X, et al. Preliminary study of magnetically controlled capsule gastroscopy for diagnosing superficial gastric neoplasia. Dig Liver Dis 2018;50(10):1041–6.
48. Liao Z, Hou X, Lin-Hu E-Q, et al. Accuracy of magnetically controlled capsule endoscopy, compared with conventional gastroscopy, in detection of gastric diseases. Clin Gastroenterol Hepatol 2016;14(9):1266–73.e1261.
49. Chen Y-Z, Pan J, Luo Y-Y, et al. Detachable string magnetically controlled capsule endoscopy for complete viewing of the esophagus and stomach. Endoscopy 2019;51(4):360–4.
50. Song J, Bai T, Zhang L, et al. Better view by detachable string magnetically controlled capsule endoscopy for esophageal observation: a retrospective comparative study. Dis Esophagus 2020;33(4):doz104.
51. Singeap A-M, Stanciu C, Trifan A. Capsule endoscopy: the road ahead. World J Gastroenterol 2016;22(1):369–78.

52. Wang L, Zhang G, Luo JC, et al. Wireless spectroscopic compact photonic explorer for diagnostic optical imaging. Biomed Microdevices 2005;7(2):111–5.

53. Ray K. Endoscopy: tethered capsule endomicroscopy of the oesophagus–an easy pill to swallow. Nat Rev Gastroenterol Hepatol 2013;10(3):129.

54. Sharma VK. The future is wireless: advances in wireless diagnostic and therapeutic technologies in gastroenterology. Gastroenterology 2009;137(2):434–9.

55. Seibel EJ, Carroll RE, Dominitz JA, et al. Tethered capsule endoscopy, a low-cost and high-performance alternative technology for the screening of esophageal cancer and Barrett's esophagus. IEEE Trans Biomed Eng 2008;55(3):1032–42.

56. Gora MJ, Sauk JS, Carruth RW, et al. Tethered capsule endomicroscopy enables less invasive imaging of gastrointestinal tract microstructure. Nat Med 2013; 19(2):238–40.

57. Stipho S, Tharalson E, Hakim S, et al. String capsule endoscopy for screening and surveillance of esophageal varices in patients with cirrhosis. J Interv Gastroenterol 2012;2(2):54–60.

58. Zhang H, Morgan D, Cecil G, et al. Biochromoendoscopy: molecular imaging with capsule endoscopy for detection of adenomas of the GI tract. Gastrointest Endosc 2008;68(3):520–7.

59. Wicks T, Clain D. A guide wire for rapid jejunal biopsies with the Crosby capsule. Gut 1972;13(7):571.

60. Kong, Kyoungchul & Cha, Jinhoon & Jeon, Doyoung & Cho, Dong-il. (2005). A rotational micro biopsy device for the capsule endoscope. Proceedings of the IEEE/RSJ International Conference on Intelligent Robots and Systems. 1839 - 1843. 10.1109/IROS.2005.1545441.

61. Rathbone M, Hadgraft J, Roberts M. Modified-release drug delivery technology. CRC Press 2002;126(4):35–48.

62. Wilding n, Hirst n, Connor n. Development of a new engineering-based capsule for human drug absorption studies. Pharm Sci Technol Today 2000;3(11):385–92.

63. Whitehurst, Todd & Schulman, Joseph & Jaax, Kristen & Carbunaru, Rafael. (2009). The Bion® Microstimulator and its Clinical Applications. 10.1007/978-0-387-77261-5_8.

64. Clarke JO, Jagannath SB, Kalloo AN, et al. An endoscopically implantable device stimulates the lower esophageal sphincter on demand by remote control: a study using a canine model. Endoscopy 2007;39(1):72–6.

65. Malagelada C, De Iorio F, Azpiroz F, et al. New insight into intestinal motor function via noninvasive endoluminal image analysis. Gastroenterology 2008;135(4): 1155–62.

The Cost-Effectiveness of Video Capsule Endoscopy

Salmaan Jawaid, MD

KEYWORDS

- Video capsule endoscopy • Small bowel • Cost-effectiveness
- Acute gastrointestinal bleeding • Gastrointestinal pathology

KEY POINTS

- Video capsule endoscopy (VCE) is well tolerated and can be beneficial in the diagnosis and management of various gastrointestinal disorders.
- Its largest impact has been felt in patients presenting with small bowel bleeding and, more recently, in patients with acute gastrointestinal bleeding.
- The use of VCE in the current setting is proving to be cost-effective but likely will need continued investigation before widespread use.

INTRODUCTION

The advent of video capsule endoscopy (VCE) in the early 2000s capitalized on the growing trend of developing minimally invasive technology to help manage common medical problems. Gastroenterologists could now endoscopically evaluate the entire small bowel (SB) simply by having patients swallow a small camera pill.[1] Since its initiation, VCE's ability to diagnose SB gastrointestinal pathology, such as small intestinal bleeding, Crohn disease, celiac disease, and SB tumors, has been well documented.[2,3] With evolution in VCE technology, including the development of real-time viewing and the Suspected Blood Indicator (Given Imaging, Yokneam, Israel),[4] indications for deploying VCE continued to broaden, most importantly, for the evaluation of chronic obscure gastrointestinal bleeding (GIB)[5] and recently for the evaluation of acute nonhematemesis GIB (NHGIB) (melena, hematochezia, and guaiac-positive stool).[6] With its increasing use and current economic medical climate, evaluation of the cost-effectiveness of VCE in various clinical scenarios needs detailed examination.

COST-EFFECTIVENESS ANALYSIS
Definition

Cost-effective analysis is a type of economic analysis often used in medicine to evaluate the relative costs and outcomes (also known as *effect*) of making certain health care decisions. It is helpful when trying to compare the cost and effectiveness of 2

Gastroenterology-Advanced Endoscopy, Baylor College of Medicine, 7200 Cambridge Street, Suite 8B, MSBCM 901, Houston, TX 77030, USA
E-mail address: Salmaan.jawaid@bcm.edu

Gastrointest Endoscopy Clin N Am 31 (2021) 413–424
https://doi.org/10.1016/j.giec.2020.12.010
1052-5157/21/© 2020 Elsevier Inc. All rights reserved.

giendo.theclinics.com

different interventions to assess if the value of a new intervention justifies its cost. Optimally, a health care ecosystem would favor the strategy that is more effective but least costly. Centers for Medicare & Medicaid Services data often are used as a yardstick.

Costs

Costs typically refer to total net expenditure, including the cost of intervention, adverse events related to the intervention, and calculated cost savings from the prevention of the interested condition.[7] These costs can be calculated from prospectively collected or retrospectively collected data. These data can vary among different regions and payor systems, which can limit generalizability.

Effectiveness (Outcomes)

Effectiveness is measured in units of the desired outcome. The effectiveness, or outcome, of various interventions can be compared with by assessing intervention achieves the desired outcome more effectively.

Incremental Cost-Effectiveness Ratio

Often, a new strategy or intervention is more effective than the standard but incurs more costs. How should a health care decision maker interpret these results and decide on implementation? Experts in the US Public Health Service, who have created standards for assessment of cost-effective analysis, recommend that cost-effectiveness studies use quality-adjusted life years (QALYs) as 1 outcome, because they reflect the value of implementing a new health care strategy despite increased costs.[8]

The incremental cost-effectiveness ratio is calculated by dividing the difference in cost of performing the intervention by the difference in outcomes between both strategies. When measured in QALYs, it tells the evaluator how efficiently the new intervention can produce an additional QALY. The lower the ratio, the more efficiently the new intervention produces an additional QALY, thereby supporting its implementation. Unfortunately, the US Public Health Service has not adopted a level at which ratios lower than a specific level would persuade a decision maker to implement a specific intervention. Thus, it is up to the decision maker to compare the ratio to other well-documented ratios to decide if implementation is worth it. The US health care system generally accepts an efficient intervention if costs associated with new interventions are less than $50,000 per QALY.[9]

Modeling and Decision Tree Analysis

The calculation of costs and effectiveness in real time often is difficult due to inability to follow patients over extended period of times. Moreover, when multiple interventions and outcomes are possible, determining the most cost-effective strategy can become challenging. Computational modeling and decision tree analysis allows an evaluator to simultaneously assess the overall impact of multiple intervention using preexisting data for each individual intervention. Additionally, in modeling, patients are not exposed to various interventions, larger populations can be generated, and the desired effect can be quantified over a longer time interval that otherwise is not feasible in real time.

An example of a decision tree used in this manner is shown in **Fig. 1**. Decision trees are depicted as a flow chart composed of nodes and branches. Squares represent the decision made and circles represent chance nodes, which provide all the different possibilities after making the aforementioned decision. In the example are the effects (cost) of choosing an esophagogastroduodenoscopy (EGD) as the primary diagnostic

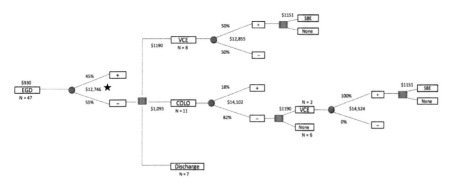

- Decision Node; ● **- Chance Node;** ★ **total incurred costs; EGD (esophagogastroduodenoscopy); COLO (Colonoscopy),**
VCE (Video capsule endoscopy); SBE (small bowel enteroscopy)

Fig. 1. Overall costs and decision flow of primary EGDs in NHGIB patients admitted to the floor. (*Adapted from* Jawaid S, Maranda L, Marya N, Cave DR. A cost utilization analysis of non-hematemesis GIB diagnostic strategies. Manuscript submitted; with permission).

modality in patients presenting with NHGIB. When an EGD is chosen, the chances it will be nondiagnostic (negative) or diagnostic (positive), based on previously identified data, are 55% and 45%, respectively. If the EGD is positive, the decision tree is completed because the desired outcome of obtaining a diagnosis has been achieved. If the EGD is negative, then a decision needs to be made on which procedure to perform next. In the example, the patient can be discharged, can undergo a colonoscopy, or can undergo a VCE. The flow chart continues like this until no more decisions need to be made and the patient has completed the work up for NHGIB. Costs with making each decision are noted at each interval. The total incurred cost associated with choosing an EGD as the primary treatment modality then is noted with a star and valued at $12,746.

In this type of modeling, values can be changed to assess variations in costs if outcomes were altered. For example, in **Fig. 2** are the effects of increasing the diagnostic yield (or positive rate) of choosing EGD as the primary diagnostic modality while keeping the diagnostic yield of other primary chosen procedures constant. If the diagnostic yield of EGD is 68% or greater, it will incur less cost than a primary VCE, as long as the diagnostic yield of VCE remains constant. For the decision maker, this means that as long as the diagnostic yield of EGD is less than 68%, it will be more costly to perform an EGD as the primary treatment modality compared with the VCE. This makes sense clinically, because a higher diagnostic yield of EGD equates to less need for further costly nondiagnostic procedures.

VIDEO CAPSULE ENDOSCOPY AND INFLAMMATORY BOWEL DISEASE

Crohn disease is a chronic inflammatory condition commonly causing ulcers, fistulas, and strictures within the SB. Current therapy for Crohn disease focuses primarily on decreasing the degree of inflammation and inducing remission. Defining remission in patients with SB Crohn disease often is difficult because clinical remission often can be present even in the setting of active mucosal disease.[10] Studies have suggested endoscopic remission (mucosal healing) often is associated with better long-term outcomes, lower need for surgery, and effective cost utilization.[11] Determining mucosal healing in patients with SB Crohn disease, however, can be challenging. Ileocolonoscopy can be helpful in these scenarios because endoscopic visualization

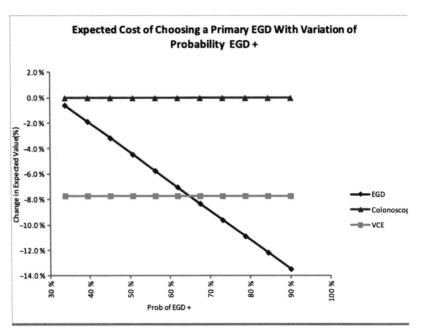

Fig. 2. Expected costs of choosing a primary EGD, with variation in probability of EGD being positive (EGD +) for patients admitted to the floor. (*Adapted from* Jawaid S, Maranda L, Marya N, Cave DR. A cost utilization analysis of non-hematemesis GIB diagnostic strategies. Manuscript submitted; with permission).

is excellent and biopsies often can be performed. Ileocolonoscopy, however, requires a bowel preparation, is invasive, and cannot assess disease activity proximal to the terminal ileum (TI), which can be involved in 16% to 65% of patients.[12,13] Cross-sectional imaging (computed tomography enterography [CTE] or magnetic resonance enterography) can be used to assess inflammation and potential complications of active inflammation (strictures, abscess, and fistulas). The former, however, is associated with radiation. The use of VCE in this scenario can evaluate the mucosal integrity of the entire SB, thereby providing a minimally invasive modality to document pan–small intestinal mucosal healing with more certainty.[12,14] A meta-analysis of 12 trials in 2010 demonstrated that VCE had superior diagnostic yields to SB radiography (SBR), CTE, and ileocolonoscopy in patients with suspected SB Crohn disease and superior diagnostic yields to SBR and CTE for patients with established SB Crohn disease.[15]

Cost-Effectiveness of Video Capsule Endoscopy in Suspected Small Bowel Crohn Disease

The algorithmic approach to the evaluation of SB Crohn disease is well aligned for a detailed cost analysis because there are multiple permutations of testing strategies for diagnosing or monitoring the disease process. Unfortunately, only a few studies exist evaluating the most cost-effective strategy. Levesque and colleagues[16] investigated whether VCE was a cost-effective diagnostic tool in the evaluation of suspected SB Crohn disease in patients with 2 previous negative test results (ileocolonoscopy and CTE/SBR). The investigators found in patients with low pretest probability (20%) of SB Crohn disease, ileocolonoscopy alone (with intubation of the TI) was the most cost-effective strategy for the diagnosis of SB Crohn disease, with increasing costs and QALYs associated with combining ileocolonoscopy with other diagnostic modalities, including VCE. In patients with high pretest (75%) probability of SB Crohn disease, the incremental cost-effectiveness ratio of ileocolonoscopy plus CTE was $54,000 per QALY gained compared with ileocolonoscopy plus CTE plus VCE, which cost more than $895,000 per QALY gained.[16] From these data, the investigators concluded, in patients with either low pretest or high pretest probability probability of SB Crohn disease and successful intubation of the TI (with negative ileocolonoscopy), that use of VCE as a third diagnostic test was not cost-effective. The same conclusion was made for patients with unsuccessful TI intubation. The investigators, however, did not evaluate the cost-effectiveness of performing VCE as the second diagnostic test after a negative ileocolonoscopy (in both successful and unsuccessful TI intubations). This limitation was addressed in a decision tree analysis comparing SBR with VCE as the second diagnostic procedure after a negative ileocolonoscopy.[17] The study demonstrated the use of VCE produced a cost savings of $291 over SBR and maintains its cost savings as long as the diagnostic yield of VCE in this setting remains at 64.1% or better. These results were reproduced by Leighton and colleagues,[18] in which demonstration of cost savings using VCE as the second diagnostic test was preserved, even after including potential costs associated with changes in therapy related to positive findings on VCE. This is no surprise because cost of initiating therapy at an earlier course of the disease may outweigh the costs associated with discovering the true extent of disease at a later time.[19,20] Moreover, the benefit of a negative VCE in these scenarios often can prove beneficial both for clinician and patient and its value is difficult to calculate from a monetary standpoint. Thus, findings or lack of findings on VCE can change therapeutic strategies directly, leading to direct improved cost utilization.

An important point regarding Levesque and colleagues' study is that increased cost associated with VCE used as a third diagnostic test was related directly to the low specificity of VCE. This low referenced specificity, however, was based primarily on 1 study by Solem and colleagues.[21] Other studies have indicated a higher specificity of VCE (>85%) for SB Crohn disease[15,22,23] and, as alluded to by Levesque and colleagues, in a 1-way sensitivity analysis, if the specificity of VCE increased, total costs per QALY gained would decrease substantially. Nevertheless, these studies highlight a point of caution: findings on VCE need to be scrutinized carefully to determine true clinical significance because labeling a patient with SB Crohn disease can have tremendous psychological and economic impact.

Based on current data on diagnostic yields and associated costs, VCE should be used in patients with suspected Crohn disease as the second diagnostic test after a negative ileocolonoscopy, as long as signs of SB strictures or obstruction are not suspected. This conclusion is supported by the American Gastroenterological Association guidelines as well.[24] In patients with very low suspicion of SB Crohn disease, use of VCE likely is not cost-effective.

Cost-Effectiveness of Video Capsule Endoscopy in Established Small Bowel Crohn Disease

The routine use of VCE in established Crohn disease appears less conflicting. Regardless of location within the SB, pathologic findings can be observed on VCE, circumventing the need for invasive testing or radiation. Only 1 cost analysis has been performed evaluating the cost-effectiveness of VCE in the monitoring of SB Crohn disease.[25] In it, Saunders and colleagues evaluated 2 scenarios: common monitoring practice, which includes ileocolonoscopy plus imaging, and direct VCE. Modeling found that over 20 years, VCE compared with common monitoring practice reduced costs ($313,367 vs $320,015, respectively), increased life expectancy (18.15 years vs 17.9 years, respectively), and increased quality of life (8.7 QALYs vs 8.0 QALYs, respectively). If implemented in 50% of patients over a 5-year period, a payer could expect a decreased cost of monitoring (–$469 mean per patient) and surgery (–$698) but increased costs for active treatments (+$717). The total savings for the payer over 5 years would be close to $36.5 million.

Future Directions

The biggest limitation of the these cost analysis studies is that they all are projections based on decision tree models. Given the continued increased use of VCE in both suspected and established SB Crohn disease, prospective cost analysis studies need to be performed. The benefit of performing a cost analysis in this way is the ability to obtain real-time costs along with real-time diagnostic yields from within the same cohort, rather than having to reference other studies involving heterogenous cohorts. Moreover, further prospective data on the true specificity of VCE for Crohn disease need to be entertained because the biggest influence on VCE costs are related to its accuracy. Determining the specificity of VCE can be accomplished with the development of validated Crohn disease scoring systems for findings on VCE, thereby minimizing interobserver variability and increasing accuracy of VCE.

VIDEO CAPSULE ENDOSCOPY AND GASTROINTESTINAL BLEEDING

By effectively visualizing gastrointestinal mucosa, use of VCE has revolutionized the ability to identify culprit bleeding lesions throughout the gastrointestinal tract. It is used most often for suspected SB bleeding, given its ability to localize the bleeding source. It has been shown to carry a diagnostic yield ranging from 40% to 60%, superior to that of push enteroscopy, CT, and angiography.[26,27] VCEs' advantage over other diagnostic procedures is its ability to tumble and take advantage of SB peristalsis by examining areas of the SB multiple times. This allows VCE to capture lesions that tend to bleed intermittently at different times (arteriovenous malformations for example) and often are found within the SB but difficult to capture while actively bleeding.[28] Moreover, VCE has the capability of being deployed without much preparation time or need for anesthesia, thereby supporting quick deployment closer to the index bleeding event with a consequent increase in diagnostic yield.[29] The cost-effectiveness of using VCE in the setting of obscure GIB and acute NHGIB is examined.

Cost-Effectiveness of Video Capsule Endoscopy Small Intestinal Bleeding

Small intestinal bleeding (occult or obscure) is defined as GIB from an unidentified source that recurs despite negative endoscopic examinations. Based on previous literature, VCE used in this scenario can increase the diagnostic yield by 25% to 50% compared with push enteroscopy or angiography.[30,31] Cost utilization analyses have demonstrated that when definitive therapy is needed, push enteroscopy is the most cost-effective strategy, whereas when localization and visual diagnosis are needed, VCE is the most cost-effective.[32] Single-balloon enteroscopy can be cost-effective as the initial strategy over initial capsule endoscopy, with a resultant incremental cost-effectiveness ratio of $20,833 per QALY gained.[33] SBE is an invasive procedure, however, and initial VCE may prove more cost-effective in the long run due to potential for fewer complications and improved utilization of resources. In a robust international study, Mueller and colleagues[34] performed a predicted cost model incorporating sensitivities and specificities of 7 controlled trials from 5 countries comparing initial VCE versus push enteroscopy. In all 5 countries, VCE was more effective and less costly than push enteroscopy when prevalence of disease was at least 30%. The most common use of VCE was at a prevalence of 50%. The findings support the use of VCE for obscure GIB, when localization of the bleeding source is needed.

Cost-Effectiveness of Video Capsule Endoscopy for Acute Nonhematemesis Gastrointestinal Bleeding

NHGIB typically is defined as acute GIB, typically presenting as melena, hematochezia, or guaiac-positive stools with anemia and no previous endoscopic work-up.[35] Unlike in patients presenting with hematemesis, where an EGD is effective in diagnosing and treating bleeding lesions, patients presenting with NHGIB can have bleeding originating from anywhere within the gastrointestinal tract, often beyond the reach of an EGD.[36] Localization of bleeding, therefore, can present a diagnostic challenge in this subset of patients with many undergoing multiple nondiagnostic endoscopic examinations.[35,36] The author's group's retrospective analyses of consecutive patients presenting to the emergency department for NHGIB demonstrated a primary EGD or colonoscopy was diagnostic in only 50% and 54% of patients, respectively, whereas a primary VCE was diagnostic in 79% of patients.[35] Expectedly, a secondary colonoscopy after a negative EGD was diagnostic only 12.5% of the time. Consequently, the author's group performed a landmark randomized controlled trial comparing initial VCE use versus standard of care in the management of acute NHGIB.[6] In it, patients were found who underwent an initial VCE were able to have localization of bleeding in 64.3% of patients compared with 31.1% in the standard-of-care arm ($P<.01$).

Although establishing initial VCE in this setting may improve diagnostic yield, it may necessitate a subsequent specific therapeutic procedure, unlike a primary diagnostic EGD or colonoscopy, which has therapeutic options. Thus, questions regarding cost-effectiveness remain. For this reason, a decision tree analysis was performed evaluating which combination of procedures would prove the most cost-effective in the complete management of patients with NHGIB (diagnostic and therapeutic) (Jawaid S, Maranda L, Marya N, et al. A cost utilization analysis of non-hematemesis GIB diagnostic strategies. Submitted for publication).[37] The diagnostic probabilities used were from a retrospective cohort already established. Findings suggested the use of VCE as the initial diagnostic test resulted in fewer incurred costs ($12,146) than an initial EGD ($12,746) or colonoscopy ($13,161). Sensitivity analysis suggested even if the diagnostic probability of an initial VCE would increase to 100%, thereby guaranteeing another therapeutic procedure, VCE use still would incur less cost ($12,445) than any other option. The author's group next performed a noninferiority cost analysis on the cohort of patients from the randomized controlled trial using actual costs derived from the hospital financial data.[36] There was no difference in total direct cost per inpatient case between both the VCE and the standard-of-care groups. Further projected analysis indicated patients could be discharged in half the amount of time within the VCE arm (0.88 days) compared with the standard-of-care arm (1.63 days) (P = .0005). Long-term cost data are pending. Conclusions from both of the author's cost analyses suggest that, in patients with NHGIB, a noninvasive initial deployment of VCE allows for more effective bleeding localization without increasing total cost associated with the management of these patients. Its use could allow for more effective cost utilization and safer outcomes, because a subsequent invasive EGD, deep enteroscopy, or colonoscopy would be used primarily for a targeted therapeutic measure rather than for diagnostic purposes.

Cost-Effectiveness of Video Capsule Endoscopy for Hematemesis or Upper Gastrointestinal Bleeding

VCE use in other areas of bleeding has been surfacing. Guidelines indicate for patients presenting with acute upper GIB (mostly manifested with hematemesis), every effort should be made to determine severity of bleeding and necessity for hospital admission for endoscopic intervention.[38] Triaging these patients, however, to allow for more efficient allocation of resources can be challenging. Multiple validated risk stratification modalities have been developed (Glasgow-Blatchford score [GBS], Rockall score, and nasogastric [NG] tube aspirate) to assist in identifying low-risk and high-risk patients.[39,40] These scores, however, have yet to be implemented practically on a regular basis and NG tube aspiration itself it not patient-friendly and does not determine severity or timing of endoscopy.[40] In addition, even in patients determined to be within the low-risk category, hospital admissions and inpatient endoscopies still are overutilized.[41] Thus, a more efficient, easily adoptable triage tool is needed.

EGD-based risk stratification is accurate but studies have suggested this often requires hospital admission and logistically can be difficult to perform quickly.[42] VCE, on the other hand, requires less allocation of resources and can be utilized in any clinical setting. Moreover, its real-time viewing capability allows visualization of the gastrointestinal tract as the capsule moves through the patient. Evidence of feasibility of VCE was best evidenced in Meltzer and colleagues'[43] study, where they demonstrated that emergency room physicians, with little background in VCE technology, could identify blood or coffee ground material accurately using real-time viewing. Ultimately, Rubin and colleagues[44] were the first to evaluate the ability of VCE to identify high-risk and low-risk stigmata lesions in patients presenting with acute upper GIB. In it, 24 patients were randomized to VCE versus standard of care. Seven of the 12 patients within the VCE arm were found to have coffee grounds, clots, red blood, or a bleeding lesion on real-time viewing. All 7 had confirmatory findings on EGD. Four of the 5 negative VCE patients underwent EGD and were found to not have high-risk stigmata lesions, correlating with findings on VCE. Time to endoscopy in the VCE-positive group was substantially shorter than standard of care (2.5 hours vs 8.9 hours, respectively; P = .0.29). The investigators concluded that live-view VCE in upper GIB patients accurately distinguished high-risk versus low-risk patients and could reduce the time to therapeutic intervention. Since then, more and more well-designed studies have reported similar findings and have determined that VCE is more accurate than clinical scoring stools and NG tube aspiration in predicting high-risk versus low-risk endoscopic stigmata for bleeding[45,46] and can be employed by both gastroenterologist and VCE-trained ER physicians.[43] But can the cost of preventing an unnecessary hospital admission outweigh the cost of deploying VCE? To answer this question, Meltzer and colleagues[47] created a model to evaluate if VCE could be a cost-effective triage tool for patients presenting with hematemesis (mild to moderate risk based on GBSs). The investigators compared 4 outcomes: (1) direct imaging via VCE, (2) risk stratification using GBSs, (3) NG tube placement, and (4) admit-all strategy. In both the low-risk and high-risk groups, direct imaging via VCE was more cost-effective and was the preferred strategy over all other strategies (cost $5691, 14.69 QALYs in low-risk group; and cost $9190, 14.56 QALYs high risk group).

SUMMARY

The technological advances in VCE mimic the evolution of its clinical indications. In an era of optimizing health care economics, use of VCE likely will continue to allow for efficient allocation of resources. Its biggest impact in the future likely will be in the management of GIB. Its implementation can allow for better localization of bleeding, thereby promoting a more efficient, targeted therapeutic option, yet still serve as a potentially cost-effective triage tool in patients presenting with GIB. Most importantly, its ease of use by both physicians and patients alike makes it application quite feasible. Further work will need to be done on development of a universal infrastructure to handle the increased use of VCE technology.

CLINICS CARE POINTS

- Video capsule endoscopy is a non-invasive, cost effective diagnostic tool for multiple gastrointestinal conditions.

DISCLOSURES

None.

REFERENCES

1. Iddan G, Meron G, Glukhovsky A, et al. Wireless capsule endoscopy. Nature 2000;405(6785):417.
2. Goel Rishi M, Kamal VP, Dean B, et al. "Video capsule endoscopy for the investigation of the small bowel: primary care diagnostic technology update." Br J Gen Pract 2014;64(620):154–6.
3. Enns RA, Hookey L, Armstrong D, et al. Clinical practice guidelines for the use of video capsule endoscopy. Gastroenterology 2017;152(3):497–514.
4. Han S, Fahed J, Cave DR. Suspected blood indicator to identify active gastrointestinal bleeding: a prospective validation. Gastroenterology Res 2018;11(2): 106–11.
5. Gerson LB, Fidler J, Cave DR, et al. ACG clinical guideline: diagnosis and management of small bowel bleeding. Am J Gastroenterol 2015;110:1265–87.
6. Marya NB, Jawaid S, Foley A, et al. A randomized controlled trial comparing efficacy of early video capsule endoscopy with standard of care in the approach to

nonhematemesis GI bleeding (with videos). Gastrointest Endosc 2019;89(1): 33–43.e4.

7. Weinstein MC, Stason WB. Foundations of cost-effectiveness analysis for health and medical practices. N Engl J Med 1977;296(13):716.

8. Gold MR, Siegel JE, Russell LB, et al. Cost-effectiveness in health and medicine. New York (NY): Oxford University Press; 1996. see p. 285 et. Seq.

9. Owens DK. Interpretation of cost-effectiveness analyses [Editorial]. J Gen Intern Med 1998;13:716–717v.

10. Klenske Entcho, Christian Bojarski, Maximilian Waldner, et al. Targeting mucosal healing in Crohn's disease: what the clinician needs to know. Therap Adv Gastroenterol 2019;12. 1756284819856865.

11. Schnitzler F, Fidder H, Ferrante M, et al. Mucosal healing predicts long-term outcome of maintenance therapy with infliximab in Crohn's disease. Inflamm Bowel Dis 2009;15(9):1295–301.

12. Samuel S, Bruining DH, Loftus EV, et al. Endoscopic skipping of the distal terminal ileum in Crohn's disease can lead to negative results from ileocolonoscopy. Clin Gastroenterol Hepatol 2012;10(11):1253–9.

13. Leighton JA, Gralnek IM, Cohen SA, et al. Capsule endoscopy is superior to small-bowel follow-through and equivalent to ileocolonoscopy in suspected Crohn's disease. Clin Gastroenterol Hepatol 2014;12(4):609–15.

14. Boroff ES, Leighton JA. The role of capsule endoscopy in evaluating both suspected and known Crohn's disease. Tech Gastrointest Endosc 2015;17(1):5–11.

15. Dionisio PM, Gurudu SR, Leighton JA, et al. Capsule endoscopy has a significantly higher diagnostic yield in patients with suspected and established small-bowel Crohn's disease: a meta-analysis. Am J Gastroenterol 2010;105(6): 1240.

16. Levesque BG, Cipriano LE, Chang SL, et al. Cost effectiveness of alternative imaging stratgeies for the diagnosis of small-bowel Crohn's disease. Clin Gastroenterol Hepatol 2010;8(3):261–7.

17. Goldfarb NI, Pizzi LT, Fuhr JP Jr, et al. Diagnosing Crohn's disease: an economic analysis comparing wireless capsule endoscopy with traditional diagnostic procedures. Dis Manag 2004;7(4):292–304.

18. Leighton JA, et al. Capsule endoscopy in suspected small bowel Crohn's disease: economic impact of disease diagnosis and treatment. World J Gastroenterol 2009;15(45):5685–92.

19. Lobo Alan, Torres Rafael Torrejon, McAlindon Mark, et al. Economic analysis of the adoption of capsule endoscopy within the British NHS. Int J Qual Health Care 2020;32(Issue 5):332–41.

20. Cohen SA, Gralnek IM, Ephrath H, et al. Capsule endoscopy may reclassify pediatric inflammatory bowel disease: a historical analysis. J Pediatr Gastroenterol Nutr 2008;47:31–6.

21. Solem CA, Loftus EV, Fletcher JG, et al. Small-bowel imaging in Crohn's disease: a prospective, blinded, 4-way comparison trial. Gastrointest Endosc 2008;68: 255–66.

22. Dubcenco E, Jeejeebhoy KN, Petroniene R, et al. Capsule endoscopy findings in patients with established and suspected small-bowel Crohn's disease: correlation with radiologic, endoscopic, and histologic findings. Gastrointest Endosc 2005; 62:538–44.

23. Jensen MD, Nathan T, Rafaelsen SR, et al. Diagnostic accuracy of capsule endoscopy for small bowel Crohn's disease is superior to that of MR enterography or CT enterography. Clin Gastroenterol Hepatol 2011;9:124–9.

24. Leighton J, Gerson LB. Use and misuse of small bowel video capsule endoscopy in clinical practice. Clin Gastroenterol Hepatol 2013;11:1224–31.
25. Saunders R, Torrejon Torres R, Konsinski L. Evaluating the clinical and economic consequences of using video capsule endoscopy to monitor Crohn's disease. Clin Exp Gastroenterol 2019;12:375–84.
26. Boal Carvalho P, Rosa B, Moreira MJ, et al. New evidence on the impact of antithrombotics in patients submitted to small bowel capsule endoscopy for the evaluation of obscure gastrointestinal bleeding. Gastroenterol Res Pract 2014;2014: 709217.
27. Buscaglia JM, Giday SA, Kantsevoy SV, et al. Performance characteristics of the suspected blood indicator feature in capsule endoscopy according to indication for study. Clin Gastroenterol Hepatol 2008;6:298–301.
28. Gunjan Deepak, Vishal S, Surinder SR, et al. Small bowel bleeding: a comprehensive review. Gastroenterol Rep (Oxf) 2014;2(4):262–75.
29. Singh A, Marshall C, Chaudhuri B, et al. Timing of video capsule endoscopy relative to overt obscure GI bleeding: implications from a retrospective study. Gastrointest Endosc 2013;77:761–6.
30. Lewis BS, Swain P. Capsule endoscopy in the evaluation of patients with suspected small intestinal bleeding: results of a pilot study. Gastrointest Endosc 2002;56:349–53.
31. Mylonaki M, Fritscher-Ravens A, Swain P. Wireless capsule endoscopy: a comparison with push enteroscopy in patients with gastroscopy and colonoscopy negative gastrointestinal bleeding. Gut 2003;52:1122–6.
32. Somsouk M, Gralnek I, Inadomi J. Management of obscure occult gastrointestinal bleeding: a cost-minimization analysis. Clin Gastroenterol Hepatol 2008;6: 661–70.
33. Gerson L, Kamal A. Cost-effectiveness analysis of management strategies for obscure GI bleeding. Gastrointest Endosc 2008;68(5):920–36.
34. Mueller E, Schwander B, Bergemann R. Cost effectiveness of capsule endoscopy in diagnosing obscure gastrointestinal bleeding. Gastrointest Endosc 2004;59(5):A138.
35. Jawaid S, Marya N, Gondal B, et al. Lower endoscopic diagnostic yields observed in non-hematemesis gastrointestinal bleeding patients. Dig Dis Sci 2018;63(12):3448–56.
36. Ibach MB, Grier JF, Goldman DE, et al. Diagnostic considerations in evaluation of patients presenting with melena and nondiagnostic esophagogastroduodenoscopy. Dig Dis Sci 1995;40(7):1459–62.
37. Jawaid S, Marya N, Hicks M, et al. Prospective cost analysis of early video capsule endoscopy versus standard of care in non-hematemesis GIB: a noninferiority study. J Med Econ 2020;23(1):10–6.
38. Barkun AN, Almadi M, Kuipers EJ, et al. Management of nonvariceal upper gastrointestinal bleeding: guideline recommendations from the international consensus group. Ann Intern Med 2019;171(11):805–22.
39. Blatchford O, MurrayWR Blatchford M. A risk score to predict needfor treatment for upper-gastrointestinal haemorrhage. Lancet 2000;356:1318–21.
40. Stanley AJ, Dalton HR, Blatchford O, et al. Multicentre comparison of the glasgow blatchford and rockall scores in the prediction of clinical end-points after upper gastrointestinal haemorrhage. Aliment Pharmacol Ther 2011;34:470–5.
41. Dulai GS, Gralnek IM, Oei TT, et al. Over-utilization of healthcare resources for low-risk patients with acute, non-variceal upper gastrointestinal hemorrhage: an historical cohort study. Gastrointest Endosc 2002;55:321–7.

42. Lee JG, Turnipseed S, Romano C, et al. Endoscopy-based triage signifi cantly reduces hospitalization rates and costs of treating upper GI bleeding: a randomized controlled trial. Gastrointest Endosc 1999;50:755–61.

43. Meltzer AC, Pinchbeck C, Burnett S, et al. Emergency physicians accurately interpret video capsule endoscopy findings in suspected upper gastrointestinal hemorrhage: a video survey. Acad Emerg Med 2013;20:711–5.

44. Rubin M, Hussain SA, Shalomov A, et al. Live view video capsule endoscopy enables risk stratification of patients with acute upper GI bleeding in the emergency room: a pilot study. Dig Dis Sci 2011;56:786–91.

45. Gutkin E, Shalomov A, Hussain SA, et al. Pillcam ESO is more accurate than clinical scoring systems in risk stratifying emergency room patients with acute upper gastrointestinal bleeding. Therap Adv Gastroenterol 2013;6:193–8.

46. Sung JJY, Tang RSY, Ching JYL, et al. Use of capsule endoscopy in the emergency department as a triage of patients with GI bleeding. Gastrointest Endosc 2016;84:907–13.

47. Meltzer AC, Ward MJ, Gralnek IM, et al. The cost-effectiveness analysis of video capsule endoscopy compared to other strategies to manage acute upper gastrointestinal hemorrhage in the emergency department. Am J Emerg Med 2014;32:823–32.

Moving?

Make sure your subscription moves with you!

To notify us of your new address, find your **Clinics Account Number** (located on your mailing label above your name), and contact customer service at:

Email: journalscustomerservice-usa@elsevier.com

800-654-2452 (subscribers in the U.S. & Canada)
314-447-8871 (subscribers outside of the U.S. & Canada)

Fax number: 314-447-8029

Elsevier Health Sciences Division
Subscription Customer Service
3251 Riverport Lane
Maryland Heights, MO 63043

*To ensure uninterrupted delivery of your subscription, please notify us at least 4 weeks in advance of move.

ELSEVIER

Printed and bound by CPI Group (UK) Ltd, Croydon, CR0 4YY

08/05/2025

01864697-0007